BONE AND JOINT INFECTIONS

BONE AND JOINT INFECTIONS

Clayton R Perry

MD

Associate Professor
Department of Orthopaedic Surgery
Washington University School of
Medicine
St Louis, Missouri
USA

MARTIN DUNITZ

First published in the United Kingdom in 1996
by Martin Dunitz Ltd, 7–9 Pratt Street, London NW1 0AE

A CIP record for this book is available from the British Library.

ISBN: 1–85317–132–8

Composition by Keyword Typesetting, Wallington, Surrey, United Kingdom
Printed and bound in Spain by Grafos, S.A. Arte Sobre paper

CONTENTS

PREFACE

To date, there has not been an inclusive text which provides an overview of the management of bone and joint infections; there are excellent texts which deal with the management of specific problems (eg, infected arthroplasties and post-traumatic osteomyelitis) or specific techniques (eg, soft tissue coverage and distraction osteogenesis), but there has been a conspicuous absence of a source which pulls these elements together. Perhaps more importantly, there is a gap between what is perceived as the area of the orthopedic surgeon and what is perceived as the area of the internist. While there are excellent texts dealing with topics such as infectious diseases, principles of antibiotic administration and immunology, these texts are not readily available to the orthopedic surgeon, are not written from the orthopedic surgeon's perspective, and apply only marginally to bone and joint infections.

The purpose of this book is to present a collection of techniques used by orthopedic surgeons and internists to manage bone and joint infections. A sketch of the theory and science behind these techniques is designed to help place them in perspective. The first chapter describes the history of the management of bone and joint infections. It is followed by chapters dealing with the basic science of orthopedic infections, ie, the microbiology, mechanism of action of antibiotics, host response to infection, and the classification of bone and joint infections. Subsequent chapters cover the laboratory and radiographic evaluation of patients with bone and joint infections and nonoperative management, ie, antibiotic administration, electrical stimulation of bone healing, and hyperbaric oxygen. Operative management is covered in three chapters – the first deals with the management of osteomyelitis, the second deals with management of infected joints and arthroplasties, and the third is a series of case reports. It is hoped that this book will lead to a better understanding of bone and joint infections, and therefore better care of patients.

I would like to acknowledge the understanding and help of my family, Monica, Clay Jr. and Kevin, during the writing and preparation of this book.

CRP

1
HISTORICAL PERSPECTIVE

The history of the management of bone and joint infections is divided into two periods: the first period ending, and the second starting, in the mid nineteenth century, when it was realized that microorganisms caused bone and joint infections.

Prior to the discovery of the microbial basis of infection

In the 4500 years of recorded history prior to the discovery of the microbial basis of infection, a number of factors retarded the advancement of medical knowledge in general and the management of bone and joint infections specifically. During this period it was not understood that there were basic principles upon which management of bone and joint infections should be based; eg, Hippocrates recommended cleansing of wounds on the one hand and on the other hand he recommended cauterization, a technique which must have resulted in large amounts of residual contaminants and necrotic tissue. One reason that the basic principles of management of bone and joint infections were not understood

is that the scientific method, ie, observations, developing a hypothesis based upon these observations, and then testing the hypothesis, was not in use. The absence of this method led to misconceptions; eg, Dupuytren, like all surgeons prior to Semmelweis, Lister and Pasteur, hypothesized that bone and joint infections were due to air being let into the body.[1] This hypothesis was probably based on valid observations of the sequelae of open fractures, but it was never tested. It was not until the end of this period that scientists like Monroe and Hunter provided a sound basis for the pathology of bone and joint infections. Their observations, along with similar observations, were the origin of the hypothesis that microbes caused infections. In addition to the absence of the scientific method there was no effective method to report results meaningfully, in such a way that future practitioners could base their management on previous work. Thus, the history of this period consists of advances made by various outstanding individuals. In many cases these advances were forgotten when the individual died, only to be rediscovered later; eg, Galen's advocacy of ligating vessels, instead of cauterizing, to obtain hemostasis was forgotten for 14 centuries until it was rediscovered by Ambroise Paré.

Prior to the discovery of the microbial basis of infection bone and joint infections were recognized as a sequela of compound fractures and dislocations. As such, their management was described in early medical texts, the oldest of which is the Edwin Smith Papyrus.[2] The Edwin Smith Papyrus was written around 3000 BC in Egypt by a man named Imhotep. Osler considered Imhotep to be "the first figure of a physician to stand out clearly from the mists of antiquity".[3] The Edwin Smith Papyrus consists of case reports organized according to the anatomical area involved. Each case has a diagnosis, prognosis, and plan of management. Among these cases are found the first descriptions of open fractures and wound infections. In general, management of open fractures consisted of splinting and application of poultices, as exemplified by Case 37, which describes the diagnosis and management of an open fracture of the humerus. "If thou examinest a man having a break in his upper arm over which a wound has been inflicted, and thou findest that break crepitates under thy fingers, thou shouldst make for him two splints; thou shouldst bind it with ymrw, and thou shouldst treat it afterward with grease, honey, and lint every day until thou knowest that he has reached a decisive point."[4]

Hippocrates (c460–c377 BC) was born into an Asclepiad family on the island of Cos off the coast of Greece. Asclepiads were followers of the god Asclepius. They were healers who practiced their trade near temples. Asclepiad methods of healing were limited to prayer and induction and interpretation of dreams. However, they kept records which were handed down from generation to generation, and thus became a basis of knowledge on which to build. Hippocrates made three major contributions to medicine. First, and most importantly, he dissociated the practice of medicine from the religious mystiscm of the Asclepiads. Second, he combined existing knowledge with his own observations and thus moved the practice of medicine towards what we consider science. Third, he demanded that physicians have high moral standards, that they not perform abortions, not commit euthanasia, and that they maintain the confidentiality of their patients.

Writings attributed to Hippocrates were collected in the fourth century BC under the rule of Ptolemy. These writings were compiled in the library of Alexandria, and are known as the Corpus Hippocraticum. The Corpus Hippocraticum was written by many authors, but the surgical books including sections dealing with the diagnosis and management of fractures and wounds was probably written by Hippocrates himself. These writings are typified by the following description of tetanus. "The master of a large ship mashed the index finger of his right hand with the anchor. Seven days later a somewhat foul discharge appeared; then trouble with his tongue – he complained that he could not speak properly. The presence of tetanus was diagnosed, his jaws became pressed together, his teeth were locked, then symptoms appeared in his neck; on the third day opisthotonus appeared with sweating. Six days after the diagnosis was made he died."[5] This is a curt, clear, accurate description of a disease which at that time was always fatal. The reader senses the author's feeling of helplessness as the symptoms progress. Hippocrates' motive in describing such cases was to relate his knowledge, not to report his successes, and, therefore, the majority of his observations are remarkably pertinent. His greatest contribution to the management of compound fractures and of wounds was to recommend splinting and the use of clean dressings. When describing the symptoms and management of wound infections Hippocrates instructed that medicated dressings should be placed around the wound, not on it. His statement that "diseases which are not cured by medicines are cured by iron, those which are not cured by iron are cured by fire, and those not cured by fire are incurable" was the primary origin of cauterization with hot oil or heated metal. The practice of cauterization resulted in enormous suffering in the ensuing 2000 years.

Alexandria was founded by Alexander the Great in 331 BC. Its library and museum soon became the center of science and medicine of the Mediterranean basin. The two most notable physicians from Alexandria were Herophilus and Erasistratus (c300 BC). These two practitioners not only dissected corpses, but, incredibly, performed vivisections on criminals. The progress in medicine made in Alexandria was recorded by two citizens of Rome, Celsus and Galen. The writings of Claudius Galen (129–199 AD) are particularly important as they relate to surgical technique. Galen described ligature of blood vessels, making it possible to amputate an extremity without having to use cauterization to obtain hemostasis. Although ligating vessels soon fell into disrepute, in favor of cautery, it was rediscovered by Ambroise Paré over 1400 years later, and has remained the standard practice. Galen also penned the expression "laudable pus", understanding that the presence of pus often was a good prognostic sign, probably because it indicated an active defense against disease.

The next 1300 years were characterized by a lack of progress in medicine and surgery. The writings of Celsus and Galen were considered to be dogma, and were not challenged. This began to change in the thirteenth and fourteenth centuries. For example, Theodoric and Henri de Mondeville, writing in this time period, opposed Galen's concept of "laudable pus" and advocated avoiding suppuration with clean dry dressings and regular irrigation of wounds with spring water.[6] The gradual enlightenment of the thirteenth and fourteenth centuries served as a spring board for Ambroise Paré, truly one of the most remarkable personalities in the history of surgery.

Ambroise Paré (1510–1590) is widely recognized for three contributions: the harmful effects of cautery; the use of ligature to obtain hemostasis; and the importance of the orientation of the fetus in obstetrics. More importantly, but less widely recognized, Ambroise Paré was one of the first surgeons to write in the vernacular, and it was he who provided the final impetus that moved the practice of surgery away from dogma toward independent thought.

The accomplishment for which Paré is most widely recognized is his condemnation of cautery in favor of hemostasis by ligature. This was based upon observations that he made when oil, which was heated and used to cauterize stumps, was not available. Paré was forced to achieve hemostasis by ligation of vessels according to the method described by Galen. He found that the stumps healed more quickly and the patients recovered more fully when hemostasis had been achieved with ligature. The practice of ligating arteries and veins following amputation instead of searing the stump became accepted worldwide. This was extremely important because amputation was the accepted treatment for open fractures and gunshots of the extremities until the early nineteenth century; eg, D. J. Larrey, a surgeon in Napoleon's army during the Russian campaign, described performing over 300 amputations within a 24 hour period.[7]

Although Paré practiced in all areas of medicine, his observations regarding fractures, dislocations, and the all too frequent sequelae of infection are remarkably clear. For example, after describing how he had sustained an open tibia fracture (he was kicked by a horse) and the initial management (digital removal of clot and loose bone fragments, reduction, and splinting) he describes his clinical course: "Even such an exquisite regimen could not protect me against the fever that seized me on the 11th day, with drainage which caused me an abscess which suppurated a long time. I believe all of this happened because of some humor retained in the part, as well as not having been able to stand having the wound tightly enough bandaged at first, as well as for some comminuted fragments separated from the ends of the bones, made both by the fracture and its reduction."[8] Paré's fracture went on to heal without any signs of infection, and he eventually walked without a limp.

A major step in the management of open fractures was taken by Pierre Desault (1738–1795). He advocated cleansing the wound and releasing tension with incisions which lengthened the wound. He called this procedure "débridement". Most surgeons today understand débridement to mean the removal of debris from a wound. In reality débridement stems from the word *desbrider*, "to unbridle", reflecting the emphasis on the release of tension.[9] This concept was popularized by Larrey and Pierre François Percy, both of whom were surgeons in Napoleon's army. Percy wrote, "The primary purpose of the operation is to change the nature of the wound, as nearly as possible, into an incised wound."[9,10] This is exactly what our goals of management are today with contaminated or infected wounds.

The pinnacle of surgical technique in this "premicrobial period" is exemplified by two surgeons, Gross and Hamilton. Gross, a respected surgical authority and professor of surgery and anatomy at the Jefferson Medical College in Philadelphia, recommended removal of sequestra, stating that "The first and most important object of the surgeon should be to expel the dead portion of the bone and thus enable nature to effect a complete and permanent cure". Following the removal of the dead bone, the extremity was splinted to decrease the possibility of fracture. Gross recommended leaving these débrided wounds open and performing frequent dressing changes.[11] In 1881, Hamilton reported filling infected bony cavities with sea sponges soaked in carbolic acid.[12] He believed that the sponge was acting as a scaffolding for capillaries, and apparently did not realize the importance of sterilizing the cavity. In his report, there is no mention of the antiseptic properties of carbolic acid. Hamilton simply states that the sponge does not have to be soaked in the carbolic acid for a "long time".

While surgical techniques were evolving, observations which would provide a basis for our understanding of bone and joint infections were being made. "Caries" of bone was first described by Alexander Monroe in 1740. He described "ulceration of osseous tissue" due to "local injury or constitutional indisposition, such as syphilis, scrofula etc."[11] John Hunter expanded upon this premise and wrote, "In

their specific diseases the bones also resemble the soft parts". However, unlike soft tissue, "if a spontaneous opening takes place it is not sufficient for a cure; therefore the trephine is often necessary; or it may be necessary to destroy the living principal in the bone and then the actual cautery will be necessary".[13] John Hunter was the first surgeon to clearly describe an involucrum and a sequestrum.

The transition into the period following the discovery of the microbial basis of infection was not smooth. Numerous surgeons for one reason or another refused to accept the principles of asepsis and antisepsis. For example, Gross, cited above for his insightful surgical technique, denied the microbial origin of osteomyelitis and therefore did not use aseptic technique. This is painfully obvious in Samuel Eakins' painting entitled "Dr. Gross' Clinic", in which the surgeon and his assistants surround an operative field. They wear street clothes, possibly having just visited an infected patient. In fact, nine years after Lister's publication in *The Lancet* of the first 11 cases of open fracture treated with antiseptic surgery, Gross wrote "Little if any faith is placed by any enlightened or experienced surgeon on this side of the Atlantic in the so-called carbolic acid treatment of Professor Lister."[14] This closed minded approach to the microbial basis of infection was prevalent at the middle and end of the nineteenth century; it slowed the acceptance of aseptic and antiseptic techniques, increased the morbidity and mortality of disease and childbirth and destroyed Ignaz Semmelweis, one of the pioneers of asepsis.

Following the discovery of the microbial basis of infection

The period following the discovery of the microbial basis of infection is further divided in two parts: the first ends and the second starts with the advent of effective antimicrobial agents.

Prior to antimicrobial agents

Three physicians opened the postmicrobial era roughly in the mid nineteenth century. They were Ignaz Semmelweis, Joseph Lister, and Louis Pasteur.

Semmelweis practiced obstetrics in Vienna at the Allgemaines Krankenhaus. Through a series of observations he proved beyond doubt that postpartum infections were spread by contact between contaminated doctors or nurses and obstetrical patients. His observations were that: patients of doctors who attended autopsies had a higher mortality rate than patients of midwives who did not attend autopsies; when doctors came directly from the autopsy room and examined postpartum patients the mortality rate was extremely high; and that the majority of women who died of postpartum sepsis had been examined on a day that an autopsy had been performed prior to their examination. His suspicions were confirmed at an autopsy of a colleague who had died of an infected scalpel wound, sustained during an autopsy of a woman who had died of postpartum infection. The organs of his colleague showed the identical changes found in women who had died of postpartum fever. Based upon these observations, Semmelweis required doctors to scrub their hands between each obstetrical examination. This lowered the postpartum mortality from 18% to 1%. Instead of being recognized for his achievements Semmelweis was condemned because of professional jealousy. His privileges were limited and his academic rank was lowered. He left Vienna and went to Budapest where he practiced his theories, again lowering the incidence of postpartum infections, and again becoming the target of personal attacks. Eventually Semmelweis was broken by the obstinate stupidity of the medical community. He was committed to an asylum where he died in 1865 of blood poisoning.[15]

Lister (1827–1912) was a professor of surgery in Glasgow in the middle of the nineteenth century. He observed that open fractures, as opposed to closed fractures, commonly developed the complication of infection. He concluded that infection following open fracture was due to invisible particles in the air, which he termed "disease dust". When Pasteur's work was brought to Lister's attention, he correlated his observations with those of Pasteur, and made the obvious connection between "disease dust" and microbes. Lister began his practice of spraying carbolic acid into the air over the patient preoperatively and intraoperatively to prevent contamination of the wound with bacteria.[16] Lister's first paper on this subject was published in *The Lancet* in 1867, and reported 11 cases of open fractures treated with his methods.[17] Lister's theories and methods were greeted with disbelief; however, the superior results achieved by those surgeons who followed his methods convinced the skeptics.

Pasteur was a remarkable man whose accomplishments included: the first descriptions of anaerobic and aerobic bacteria; pasteurization (the practice of heating wine or milk to 110°C to prevent spoiling); and active immunization for rabies. By far his most important contribution was the concept of the germ theory of disease. Lexer, in 1894, applied Pasteur's theories to the study of bone and joint infections, proving the causal role of microorganisms. He produced osteomyelitis in animals by inoculating experimentally produced fractures with microorganisms, thus fulfilling Koch's postulates.[18]

Semmelweis' practice of hand washing prior to examining a patient is rudimentary asepsis, ie, the removal of germs from the examination field. Lister's practice of spraying carbolic acid to kill germs in the air and on the patient is rudimentary antisepsis, ie, the killing of germs in the operative field. Pasteur's recognition of the role that microorganisms played in various diseases and Lexer's proof that microorganisms cause bone and joint infections explained the success of aseptic and antiseptic techniques. This led directly to the evolution of future methods of management of bone and joint infections (ie, removal of devitalized tissue and antibiotic therapy) and methods designed to prevent bone and joint infections (ie, the surgical scrub with antiseptic soap, use of surgical gowns, gloves and drapes, administration of perioperative antibiotics, and laminar air flow).[19]

The surgical management of open and infected fractures in the period prior to antimicrobial agents reached its zenith with the techniques described by Markoe and Carrel and Dakin.[20] Markoe's technique consisted: antisepsis according to Lister's technique; débridement; fracture reduction; closure of the wound over rubber catheters; immobilization of the extremity with plaster splints; and instillation of carbolic acid several times a day via the rubber catheters.[21] The technique described by Carrel and Dakin was similar to that described by Markoe, with two notable exceptions.[22] The wound was left open until it was clean, and the irrigant was sodium hypochlorite, today known as Dakin's solution.[23]

The discovery of antimicrobial agents

Despite the knowledge that microorganisms caused infection, there were no drugs that killed the microorganisms without being extremely toxic to the patient. Paul Ehrlich's search for a "magic bullet" which would kill bacteria but not harm the host was rewarded by the synthesis of arsenicals. Salversan became the standard therapy for syphilis, and for the first time patients with syphilis had a good chance of recovery.

Thirty years after Salversan the antibacterial effects of the sulfanilamides were discovered. This discovery was a direct outgrowth of Ehrlich's observation that certain dyes had an affinity for bacteria. Gerhard Domagk, the director of Bayer Laboratories, discovered that prontosil, a textile dye, was active against *streptococci* in mice. He used prontosil in patients with infections and reported his results in 1935.[24] Clinical use of prontosil dramatically improved the prog-

nosis of many infectious diseases, including osteomyelitis.[25] Chemical and clinical studies throughout the world extended the use of sulfonamides to their maximum efficacy. Trefouel, in France, showed that prontosil was altered by the body to sulfanilamide. Other work yielded a variety of derivatives of sulfanilamide, including sulfathiazole and sulfadiazine. In 1939 Domagk received the Nobel Prize for his discovery of sulfonamides.

Despite the success of synthetic dyes, it was microorganisms themselves which provided the drugs which are most frequently used in the management of infections. This group of drugs, antibiotics, is synthesized by microorganisms in the wild, presumably to decrease environmental competition. A series of publications in the early twentieth century observed that molds, fungi and higher bacteria produced substances which prevented the growth of other bacteria in their proximity. These observations culminated in a report by Fleming in 1929.[26] In this fascinating paper, Fleming reported a serendipitous discovery. He found that colonies of *Staphylococcus* grown on plates which had later become contaminated with various microorganisms were lysed around one specific contaminating organism. This organism was *Penicillin rubrum*. He grew *P. rubrum* in broth which he then filtered. He established the spectrum of activity of this "mold broth filtrate" which he called penicillin, and he noted its lack of systemic toxicity in rabbits. Fleming went on to advocate the use of penicillin, not systemically, but as a local antiseptic to be applied to dressings. In 1941 Florey and Chain studied the clinical usefulness of systemic penicillin and began to synthesize it in quantity.

Investigators studied antibiotics produced by other microorganisms. Waksman obtained streptomycin from the organism *Streptomyces griseus* in 1944. Streptomycin was later used with isoniazid to treat tuberculosis, a previously untreatable disease. Other strains of *Streptomyces* yielded aureomycin and chloromycetin, signaling that the age of antibiotics had arrived.

At the present time, the use of antibacterial agents in combination with sound surgical principles forms the basis of the management of bone and joint infections. New antimicrobials have been and will continue to be developed with differing spectra of activity. Microorganisms will continue to develop resistance, leaving us with the question, will technology be able to keep pace with the appearance of resistant strains, or will we in essence return to the period before antimicrobial agents were available?

References

1   Dupuytren G (1777–1835) Clark, FLG (1811–1892. tr, ed), *On the injuries and diseases of bones: being selections from the collected edition of the clinical lectures of Baron Dupuytren* (Syndenham Society: London 1847) Part II Chapter IV.

2   Pickett JC, A short historical sketch of osteomyelitis, *Ann Med Hist* (1935) 7:183–191.

3   Osler W, *The evolution of modern medicine* (Yale University Press: New Haven 1921).

4   Breasted JH, *The Edwin Smith Surgical Papyrus*. Published in facsimile and hieroglyphic transliteration with translation and commentary in two volumes (The University of Chicago Press: Chicago 1930).

5   Hippocrates, Adams F (tr), *The genuine works of Hippocrates* (Williams & Wilkins: Baltimore 1939).

6   Garrison FH, *An introduction to the history of medicine*, 4th edn (WB Saunders: Philadelphia 1929).

7   Larrey DJ (1766–1842), Mercer JC (tr), *Surgical memoirs of the campaigns of Russia, Germany and France* (Carey and Lea: Philadelphia 1832).

8   Paré A, *Case reports and autopsy records*, compiled and edited by Wallace B. Hamby, translated from JP Malgaignes's Oeuvres complètes d'Ambroise Paré, Paris 1840 (Charles C. Thomas: Springfield, Illinois 1960).

9   Peltier LF, *Fractures: a history and iconography of their treatment* (Norman: San Francisco 1990).

10 Percy PF, *Manuel du chirurgien a l'Armee; ou Instrouction de chirurgie militaire* (Mequignon: Paris 1792).

11 Gross SD, *The anatomy and physiology of diseases of the bones and joints* (Grigg: Philadelphia 1830).

12 Hamilton DJ, On sponge-grafting, *J Anat Physiol* (1881) 27: 385–413.

13 Hunter J, Palmer JF, *Lectures on the principles of surgery* (Haswell, Barrington, and Haswell: London 1835).

14 Rutkow IM, *Surgery: an illustrated history* (Mosby: St Louis 1993).

15 Lyons AS, Petrucelli RJ, *Medicine: an illustrated history* (HN Abrams: New York 1978).

16 Cheyne Sir WW, *Lister and his achievements* (Longmans, Green: London 1925).

17 Lister J, On a new method of treating compound fractures, abscesses etc. with observation on the condition of suppuration, *Lancet* (1867) i:326–9, 357–9, 387–9, 507–9; ii: 95–6.

18 Lexer E VIII, Zur experimentellen erzeugung osteomyelitischer herde, *Arch Klin Chir* (1894) 48:181–200.

19 Ravitch M, *A century of surgery 1980–1990* (JB Lippincott: Philadelphia 1981).

20   Keen WW, *The treatment of war wounds* (WB Saunders: Philadelphia 1917).

21   Markoe TM, "Through drainage" in the treatment of open wounds, *Am J Med Sci* (1880) **158**:305–45.

22   Carrel A, Traitment abortif de l'infection dex plaies, *Bull Acad Med Paris* (1915) **74**:361–368.

23   Dakin HD, On the use of certain antiseptic substances in the treatment of infected wounds, *BMJ* (1915) **ii**:318–320.

24   Domagk G, Ein Beitrag zur Chemotherapie der bakteriellen Infektionen, *Dt Med Wschr* (1935) **61**: 250–253.

25   Hoyt WA, Davis EE, van Buren G, Acute hematogenous staphylococcus osteomyelitis: treatment with sulfathiazole without operation, *JAMA* (1941) **117**:2043–2050.

26   Fleming A, On the antibacterial action of cultures of a penicillium, with special reference to their use in the isolation of *B. influenzae*, *Br J Exp Path* (1929) **10**:226–238.

2
BASIC SCIENCE

This chapter reviews the microbiology, mechanism of action of antibiotics and the host response to infection.

Microbiology

Bacteria: their structure, growth, and virulence

Bacteria, along with blue-green algae, represent the simplest living organisms. As a group these organisms are called the procaryotes. All other living organisms (excluding viruses) are eucaryotes. Procaryotes are distinguished by the absence of a nucleus and mitochondria, and the presence of a unique circular DNA. There are significant differences between the structure of bacterial and eucaryotic ribosomes and lipids. Because bacteria do not have a nucleus the ribosomes are near the DNA. Therefore, bacteria can synthesize proteins directly from messenger RNA, thus linking transcription with translation and speeding the process of protein synthesis. Eucaryotes, on the other hand, must transport the messenger RNA through their nuclear membrane to the ribosomes in the cytoplasm. This is a more difficult process but allows better control of growth.

Bacteria protect their cytoplasm with a cell wall. We classify bacteria according to their type of cell wall as being: Gram positive; Gram negative; or acid fast. Gram positive denotes the retention of a purple iodine dye by the bacterial cell wall when it is washed in alcohol. Gram negative cell walls do not retain the dye when they are washed in alcohol. The cell walls of acid fast bacteria retain dye even when washed with dilute acid solutions.

Gram positive organisms are encapsulated in a cell wall composed of sugars which are cross-linked by peptides. This polymer is called murein. Although there are subtle differences in the composition of murein between different bacteria, the overall structure is similar. The cell wall prevents bacteria from bursting when exposed to media of a lower osmotic pressure than their cytoplasm. The numerous layers of murein are hydrophilic and prevent the passage of hydrophobic molecules into the cytoplasm. It is the hydrophilic nature of the murein molecule that is responsible for the retention of dye and the Gram positive label.

Gram negative bacteria have a murein cell wall and in addition they have a second, outer membrane composed of phospholipids and bacterial lipopolysaccharides. This outer membrane is hydrophobic and contains protein pores which allow the passage of charged molecules such as amino acids. It is this outer, hydrophobic membrane that prevents the dye from reaching the murein and results in the gram negative label. The space between the murein cell wall and the outer membrane is the periplasmic space. It contains the periplasm, a gel like solution of degradative enzymes and binding proteins that "soak up" amino acids and sugars. In addition, the periplasm contains enzymes which are active against various antibiotics. The ability to concentrate enzymes which degrade antibiotics in this periplasmic space makes gram negative bacteria more resistant to these antibiotics (eg, the penicillins).

The third type of cell wall occurs in acid fast bacteria. These organisms form a thick cell wall composed largely of waxes, complexed with sugars and peptides. This layer isolates the bacteria not only from harsh chemicals and changes in osmotic pressure but also from nutrients; therefore acid fast bacteria grow slowly. They are called acid fast because when they are heated the waxes in the cell wall will bind to dyes. These dyes are retained even when the cells are washed with dilute acid solutions.

Whether they are Gram positive, Gram negative or acid fast, microorganisms are divided into two groups – pathogenic and nonpathogenic. Pathogenic bacteria have characteristics which cause disease; eg, *Clostridium tetani* synthesizes the exotoxin tetanospasmin, which causes the disease tetanus. Nonpathogenic organisms are those organisms which we encounter daily on our skin, in our digestive tract, etc, that do not cause disease. Pathogenicity is not always species specific. For example, only certain strains of *Staphylococcus aureus* synthesize the exotoxin responsible for toxic shock syndrome. Although toxic shock syndrome was originally described as being the result of vaginal colonization, case

reports by Irvine et al and others have documented that postoperative orthopedic infections caused by these strains of *Staphylococcus aureus* are also associated with toxic shock syndrome.[1] The distinction between pathogenic and nonpathogenic is blurred in patients with compromised resistance. Compromised resistance can be systemic, eg, acquired immunodeficiency, or local, eg, a metallic implant or hypovascularity.

Different species or strains of pathogenic bacteria differ widely in their ability to cause disease. The term virulence refers to the degree of pathogenicity, and represents the balance between the reproducing bacteria and the defenses of the host. Bacteria reproduce by division; therefore, the maximum rate of growth is exponential, regardless of the size of the inoculum. Active host defenses slow the rate of bacterial growth. Therefore, it takes longer to reach the threshold number of bacteria at which symptoms of infection become evident if the initial inoculum is small and if host defenses are active. Virulence is quantified in the laboratory as the number of organisms which when injected into a group of animals will result in 50% of the animals dying. This measurement is called lethal dose 50, or LD50.

The study of microbial ecology yields valuable insights into how infections occur (Fig 2.1) In the aquatic environment, *Pseudomonas aeruginosa* and many other species of bacteria exist in one of two phases, planktonic swarmer cells, or surface adherent microcolonies.[2] The microcolonies exist in a layer of glycocalyx, which affords protection from predators. The swarmer cells are released from microcolonies. Their role is to attach to and colonize new surfaces; however, unprotected by glycocalyx most swarmer cells are rapidly killed. The initial attraction of bacteria to the surface is based upon the physical characteristics of the bacterium, the fluid interface and the surface substrate. Electrical charges of the bacteria and the substrate, van der Waal's forces, and hydrophobic forces all promote or inhibit the initial reversible binding.[3] Following the initial binding, the bacteria synthesize

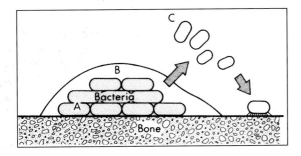

Figure 2.1

Schematic drawing of a microcolony of bacteria (A) covered with a protecting layer of glycocalyx (B). Planktonic swarmer cells are given off by the colony (C). The majority of the planktonic cells are killed; however, some manage to attach to a surface, where they form new colonies.

proteinaceous adhesions to specific sites on the surface.[4] These sites, or receptors, may be glycoprotein surface residues, or specific molecules found in cells (eg, collagen[5], fibronectin[3], and laminin, which is found in basement membranes[6]).

The analogous situation exists in bone and joint infections. Unattached bacteria are somehow introduced to, adhere to, and then colonize the surface of an implant or necrotic bone. They form microcolonies, which are protected from host defense factors by a layer of glycocalyx. Mobile swarmer cells are released continually from these microcolonies. In most cases host defenses rapidly kill these swarmer cells and the spread of infection is via growth and direct extension of the microcolonies. Occasionally spread is hematogenous via the swarmer cells. This is more common in immunocompromised patients, or when the inoculum of swarmer cells is so large that it overwhelms the host defences (eg, in burn patients). Gristina and Costerton have found that over half of prosthesis centered orthopedic infections are caused by glycocalyx producing adherent organisms, indicating that the above model applies to most, but not all, orthopedic infections.[7]

Antibiotic resistance

Multiple factors determine the relative antimicrobial activity of a drug against a specific microorganism. These factors are antibiotic dependent (ie, ability of the antibiotic to penetrate the infected area, and activity of the antibiotic against bacteria given a specific level of metabolism) or bacteria dependent (ie, are the bacteria free floating or adherent, and have they developed mechanisms of resistance?).[8,9]

Antibiotic dependent factors

Penetration of antibiotics into a given area is not uniformly predictable. Penetration often depends upon the pH or osmolality of the environment.[10,11] Therefore, a given antibiotic may not be effective in abscesses or around necrotic tissue. The effectiveness of the antibiotic may be dependent upon the metabolic activity of the microbe, with more actively growing and dividing bacteria being more susceptible. This is particularly true of bactericidal antibiotics, which work by causing the bacteria to synthesize meaningless substrates (eg, aminoglycosides and vancomycin).

Bacteria dependent factors

Resistance to antibiotics is either due to colonization of surfaces, or acquired heritable changes in the metabolism of the bacteria. Microbes which are adherent to surfaces have an increased resistance to antibiotics. In in vitro studies Naylor et al have shown that antibiotic susceptibility of floating and adherent bacteria differs.[12] Webb et al have shown that adherent *Staphylococcus aureus* colonies have minimal bactericidal concentrations 50 to 100 times higher than floating bacteria.[13] Merritt et al have shown that antibiotic penetration of the glycocalyx layer, which covers adherent bacteria, is limited.[14] They thus provide a partial explanation for the increase in resistance to antibiotics seen in adherent bacteria. That more is involved than just decreased antibiotic penetration of glycocalyx has been shown by Naylor et al, Oga et al, and Webb et al.[12,13,15] These investigators have shown that antibiotic resistance is associated not only with surface colonization but also the type of biomaterial substrate. There is a consistent pattern of an increase in antibiotic resistance of bacteria cultured on: stainless steel, polymethyl methacrylate (PMMA), and bone, with bacteria grown on stainless steel being least resistant. This substrate dependent resistance is seen in both slime-producing and non-slime-producing bacteria and is therefore independent of glycocalyx production. It may be attributable to changes in the metabolism of surface adherent organisms in a specific biomaterial microclimate. Petty et al studied the effect of the substrate on the incidence of infection in a dog model.[16] They found that PMMA which polymerized in vivo (ie, it was implanted when in its doughy state) increased the susceptibility to infection more than stainless steel, polyethylene, or polymerized PMMA. They reasoned that the increased susceptibility to infection is due to heat necrosis of surrounding tissue and to the methylmethacrylate monomer. Work published earlier by Petty indicates that the PMMA monomer decreases: the effectiveness of bacterial inhibiting serum factors; the activity of the complement sequence; production of chemotactic factors; migration of polymorphonuclear leukocytes; and phagocytosis and killing of bacteria by polymorphonuclear leukocytes.[17-20] Based upon these studies, it is clear that in vitro adherent bacteria are more resistant to antibiotics than floating bacteria. In many cases adherent bacteria are resistant to levels of antibiotics well above permissible therapeutic levels. This resistance is in part due to glycocalyx production and in part due to the substrate to which the bacteria adhere.

That the theoretical increased resistance due to bacterial adherence is clinically significant in bone and joint infections is supported by data reported by Gristina et al, and Marrie and Costerton.[21-22] In both of these reports an electron microscope was used to scan material obtained from surgical débridement of bone and joint infections. Both investigators found extensive colonies of adherent bacteria. Gristina found that "the infecting bacteria grew in coherent microcolonies in an adherent biofilm so extensive it often obscured the infected bone surfaces". Gristina et al go on to point out that the bacteria shed from these microcolonies (presumably the bacteria cultured from pus or drainage) may not be representative of those remaining in the microcolony. In a follow-up report Gristina and Costerton examined an infected prosthesis with an electron microscope.[7] They found that while wound swabs often identified only one organism, the morphology of the bacteria colonizing the surfaces of the prosthesis indicated a polymicrobial infection. These studies underscore the necessity of obtaining tissue and debris for culture, not just fluid, in order to identify accurately all species of the infecting organisms and their sensitivities to antibiotics.

Most significantly, microbes have the ability to develop, or acquire, resistance to an antibiotic. True antibiotic resistance is heritable, reflecting a change in the genetic material of the bacteria. The classic case of antibiotic resistance occurred with *Staphylococcus aureus* and penicillin G. Shortly after the introduction of penicillin G, resistant strains of *Staphylococcus aureus* appeared. Their frequency has increased so that over 80% of both hospital and community acquired strains of *Staphylococcus aureus* are no longer sensitive to penicillin G. Emergence of resistance in other species has also occurred. In 1974 a strain of penicillinase producing gonococcus emerged. These strains are resistant to high doses of penicillin G and have spread throughout the world. Likewise strains of *Streptococcus pneumoniae* resistant to penicillin G, which first appeared in 1978, are now common.

The mechanism of acquired resistance can be broken down into two broad areas: decreased penetration of the antibiotic into the bacterial cell; and decreased effectiveness of the antibiotic on its final target, a type of "end organelle resistance". Decreased penetration of antibiotic into the bacterial cell may be due to enzymes on the cell surface that inactivate the drug, or an impermeable cell membrane that prevents the antibiotic from entering. Some antibiotics are dependent upon the cell to transport them through its cell wall. And organisms may become resistant by simply not synthesizing these transport systems.[23] Each class of drug has unique sites of action. Acquired resistance can be explained by modifications in these targets, ie, modification of the ribosome so that it no longer will bind with the antibiotic. The emergence and transmission of these resistance factors is due to mutation, transduction, or conjugation.

Mutations occur naturally in all large populations. Some result in small numbers of organisms being resistant to a specific antibiotic. The presence of the antibiotic in the media selects for organisms with these mutations and they multiply while sensitive strains are eradicated. The mutational changes that confer resistance to a drug may increase or decrease the pathogenicity of the microorganism. For example, strains of *Staphylococcus aureus* that develop resistance to rifampin also produce less catalase and are less virulent than nonresistant strains.[24] On the other hand, methicillin resistant *Staphylococcus aureus* and *Staphylococcus epidermidis* are more virulent than nonresistant strains.

Transduction occurs when genetic material is transported from one bacteria to another via plasmids or bacteriophages (a virus that infects bacteria). Transduction is particularly important in the transfer of resistance to: penicillin (via beta-lactamase); erythromycin; tetracycline; and chloramphenicol among strains of *Staphylococcus aureus*.

Conjugation involves the passage of resistant genes of R factors between bacteria via direct contact. Conjugation is a phenomenon limited almost exclusively to Gram negative bacilli and can occur between different species of bacteria, eg, *Shigella* and *Escherichia coli*. This is an extremely important mechanism for spread of resistance to multiple drugs. Conjugation was first recognized in Japan in 1959 following an outbreak of *Shigella flexneri* dysentery which was resistant to four different classes of antibiotics.[25]

Antibiotics

This section covers the classification of antibiotics, their pharmacokinetics and therapy with multiple antibiotics.

Classification of antibiotics

Antibiotics are defined as chemical substances produced by various microorganisms (bacteria, fungi, or actinomycetes) that suppress the growth of other microorganisms and may kill them. Many antibiotics are now modified synthetically or synthesized *de novo*. Antibiotics are classified according to: their spectrum of activity; their chemical structure; or their mechanism of action.[8,26–28] I have found that classifying antibiotics on the basis of their mechanism of action is the most useful and meaningful method. There are six basic mechanisms by which antibiotics kill or inhibit microorganisms: inhibition of bacterial cell wall formation; increasing cell membrane permeability; ribosomal inhibition; binding to the 30 S ribosomal subunit, causing it to misread RNA; interference with DNA metabolism; and antimetabolites.

Cell wall antibiotics

These antibiotics destroy cell walls either by inhibiting the synthesis of cell wall components or by activating enzymes that disrupt the cell wall. Included in this group are: the penicillins; cephalosporins; vancomycin; and bacitracin. The penicillins and cephalosporins block the transpeptidase enzyme that is responsible for the final cross-linking of polysaccharide molecules in the bacterial cell wall. This enzyme is on the outer surface of the cytoplasmic membrane and therefore these antibiotics do not have to penetrate the cell to be effective. Vancomycin and bacitracin on the other hand inhibit cell wall formation by binding to cell wall precursors and therefore must penetrate the cell to be effective.

Penicillin G is the natural penicillin. It has a half-life of only 30 minutes owing to rapid excretion by the kidneys. Penicillin is inactivated by the enzyme beta-lactamase. The semisynthetic penicillins (eg, methicillin and oxacillin) are usually active against beta-lactamase producing *Staphylococcus aureus*. Cloxacillin and dicloxacillin are oral semisynthetic penicillins. Ampicillin, amoxicillin, and carbenicillin are not resistant to beta-lactamase, but are active against numerous Gram negative bacilli. Both ampicillin and amoxicillin can be administered orally. Carbenicillin and ticarcillin are particularly effective against *Pseudomonas aeruginosa* and *Proteus*. Mezlocillin and piperacillin are known as extended spectrum penicillins. They have a spectrum of activity similar to that of ticarcillin, but are more active against *Haemophilus influenzae* and *Bacteroides fragilis*. Mezlocillin and piperacillin act in synergy with the aminoglycosides against *Pseudomonas*.

Cephalosporins are divided into first, second, and third generations. First generation cephalosporins include: cephalothin; cephradine; cephapirin; and cefazolin. Of these the most frequently used is cefazolin. It has a longer half-life than other first generation cephalosporins but is more sensitive to beta-lactamase than other first generation cephalosporins.[29,30] First generation cephalosporins are used primarily as antistaphylococcal agents; however they are also active against *Streptococcus*, *E. coli*, *Klebsiella* and *Proteus mirabilis*. Second generation cephalosporins have an increased spectrum of activity against Gram negative organisms.

Second generation cephalosporins include: cefoxitin; cephamandole; cefotetan; cefuroxime; and cefonicid. Cefoxitin and cefotetan are the most frequently used.[31] In general, second generation cephalosporins have greater Gram negative coverage, but are less active against *Staphylococcus* than first generation cephalosporins. Cefoxitin and cefotetan are more active against anaerobic organisms than other first and second generation cephalosporins.

Third generation cephalosporins include: cefotaxime; ceftazidime; ceftriaxone; and cefoperazone. Ceftazidime and ceftriaxone are the most frequently used. In general, third generation cephalosporins are more active against Gram negative organisms, but less active against Gram positive organisms than first generation cephalosporins. Ceftriaxone is an exception, as it is active against Gram positive organisms, with the exception of enterococci and many Gram negative organisms, but it is not active against *Pseudomonas aeruginosa*. Ceftazidime, on the other hand, is extremely active against *Pseudomonas aeruginosa*, and is often the drug of choice against this organism.

Other antibiotics that inhibit formation of the bacterial cell wall are aztreonam, imipenem, vancomycin and bacitracin. Aztreonam is active against Gram negative organisms only. It has no activity against anaerobic or Gram positive organisms.

Imipenem has perhaps the broadest spectrum of activity. It is active against Gram positive and Gram negative bacilli, including *Pseudomonas aeruginosa*, and anaerobic organisms. Its use has been limited by superinfection with resistant organisms and by neurologic toxicity resulting in seizures.

Vancomycin is active against Gram positive organisms. It is used primarily against methicillin resistant *Staphylococcus aureus* and *epidermidis*, and when the patient has a history of hypersensitivity to the penicillins or cephalosporins.[32] For bone and joint infections vancomycin is administered intravenously as it is not absorbed through the gastrointestinal tract. Its administration results in phlebitis; therefore, if an extended course is anticipated a central line should be inserted. Vancomycin can be administered orally for *Clostridium difficile* infections of the intestine.

Bacitracin is used locally for wound irrigation; it is not used systemically.

The most frequent complication of administration of antibiotics from this group is a severe hypersensitivity reaction. This is particularly true with the penicillins and cephalosporins. An allergy to one penicillin indicates a possible allergy to all penicillins and cephalosporins. Interstitial nephritis can be caused by penicillins, especially methicillin. Nephritis is initially indicated by eosinophilia and an increasing BUN and it may culminate in complete cessation of renal function. Ticarcillin, mezlocillin, and piperacillin can cause sodium loading and increase the bleeding time secondary to platelet dysfunction. Cephalosporins, in particular cefamandole, may cause platelet dysfunction and increased bleeding time. Imipenem is associated with neurologic toxicity and seizures. Too rapid administration of vancomycin may result in "redman syndrome". Administration of vancomycin with an aminoglycoside may result in renal eighth nerve or toxicity. Administration of vancomycin alone is associated with a low incidence of toxicity.

Cell membrane antibiotics

These antibiotics affect cell membrane permeability, allowing leakage of intracellular contents from the cell. Included in this group are: polymyxin; nystatin; and, amphotericin. Nystatin and amphotericin are antifungal agents that bind to sterols in the cell membrane, thus increasing permeability. Nystatin is used topically and amphotericin is used systemically. Administration of the latter invariably results in some nephrotoxicity.

Ribosomal inhibitors

These antibiotics bind to bacterial ribosomes and cause reversible inhibition of protein synthesis. These blocks to protein synthesis do not kill the cell, but prevent it from multiplying. Therefore, this group of antibiotics is bacteriostatic. Once the antibiotic is eliminated viable bacteria will resume growth and reproduction. Included in this group are: tetracycline; chloramphenicol; and the macrolide antibiotics (erythromycin and clindamycin).

Tetracyclines block the binding of transfer RNA-amino acid complexes to the ribosomes. Chloramphenicol allows transfer RNA-amino acid complexes to bind to ribosomes, but blocks the linking of the amino acid to the polypeptide chain. Tetracycline is seldom used today for bone and joint infections because of the emergence of resistant strains of bacteria. It remains useful in the management of brucellosis and actinomycosis. Complications include dental staining, bone lesions, photosensitivity and enterocolitis.

Chloramphenicol is a broad spectrum antibiotic with activity against Gram negative bacilli and Gram positive cocci. It can be useful in patients with penicillin hypersensitivity or renal failure (it is excreted by the liver). Fatal idiosyncratic aplastic anemia occurs in one in 40,000 cases. Reversible anemia may also occur.

Erythromycin is active against *Staphylococcus aureus* and effective in patients with penicillin hypersensitivity. Because it is bacteriostatic it should not be used in septic patients. It has few complications, the most common being cholestatic jaundice.

Clindamycin is active against all anaerobes, including *Bacteroides fragilis*, and most Gram positive cocci, the exception being enterococci. Clindamycin's effectiveness against *B. fragilis* is important. *B. fragilis* is a fecal organism and therefore very common.[33] Unlike most other anaerobes *B. fragilis* is not sensitive to penicillin. The most common complication of clindamycin administration is pseudomembranous colitis due to *Clostridium difficile*. Clindamycin must be administered intravenously or orally as it results in subcutaneous abscesses if given intramuscularly.

Antibiotics which bind to the 30 S ribosomal subunit

These agents bind to the 30 S ribosomal subunit and cause misreading of messenger RNA, resulting in the production of abnormal peptides. The accumulation of these peptides causes cell death; therefore, these antibiotics are bactericidal. Included in this group are the aminoglycosides: streptomycin; gentamicin; tobramycin; amikacin; and neomycin. These antibiotics are toxic and it is imperative to monitor peak and trough levels to prevent renal and eighth nerve toxicity. Aminoglycosides are used primarily against Gram negative bacilli. They are active against Gram positive organisms, but are seldom used because of their toxicity. Gentamicin, tobramycin, and amikacin are administered intravenously, via an antibiotic pump, or in PMMA-antibiotic beads. Gentamicin, tobramycin, and amikacin act synergistically with mezlocillin and piperacillin against many strains of *Pseudomonas aeruginosa*. Amikacin has a lower incidence of induced tolerance and there are fewer strains of resistant *Pseudomonas* to it. than to the other aminoglycosides. Neomycin is used topically in creams or in wound irrigation. Streptomycin is administered intramuscularly, most frequently to treat mycobacterium tuberculosis infections. It has significant eighth nerve toxicity.

Antibiotics which affect nucleic acid metabolism

These antibiotics interfere with transcription and translation of bacterial DNA. There are few antibiotics in this group, presumably because the bio-

chemistry of transcription in bacteria is so similar to that of the human cell that there is not a favorable therapeutic index. This group includes: rifampin; the quinolones; and metronidazole. Rifampin inhibits bacterial DNA dependent RNA polymerase, thus blocking synthesis of RNA. It can also inhibit mitochondrial DNA dependent RNA polymerase, resulting in hepatotoxicity.

The quinolones include nalidixic acid and the fluoroquinolones: ciprofloxacin; lomefloxacin; and norfloxacin. They inhibit the enzyme DNA gyrase. Nalidixic acid and norfloxacin are used for urinary tract infections only. The fluoroquinolones are usually administered orally, although recently intravenous preparations have also become available. Ciprofloxacin is the most commonly used fluoroquinolone in the management of bone and joint infections.[34] It has an extended spectrum of activity, in particular against organisms otherwise sensitive to antibiotics that must be administered intravenously (ie, Gram negative organisms and methicillin resistant *Staphylococcus*). Mader et al compared administration of ciprofloxacin with administration of nafcillin, clindamycin, and gentamicin in the management of chronic osteomyelitis.[26] They found that there was no difference in incidence of suppression of infection and that there were no clinically significant side effects to either regimen. The authors caution that indiscriminate use of ciprofloxacin results in the "rapid emergence of resistant species". This study indicates that use of these antibiotics potentially can shorten hospital stays and decrease the cost of home antibiotic therapy.

Toxicity of fluoroquinolones includes: agitation when they are administered along with caffeine; gastrointestinal symptoms; fungal overgrowth in the groin and axilla; and skin photosensitivity. Patients should be warned about photosensitivity in particular, as it can result in severe burns.

Metronidazole is a reducing compound that forms oxygen radicals. These oxygen radicals are toxic to anaerobic organisms which lack the protective enzymes superoxide dismutase and catalase. The oxygen radicals cause loss of the helical structure of DNA and breakage of DNA strands. This is an extremely useful drug against anaerobic organisms. Toxicity is rare and includes pseudomembranous colitis, and occasionally neurologic symptoms.

Antimetabolites

Antimetabolites are structural analogues of natural metabolites. These analogues substitute for metabolic substrates and block further synthesis of products necessary for replication, ie, trimethoprim and the sulfonamides block folic acid synthesis. The antimetabolites are bacteriostatic. Included in this group are: trimethoprim; sulfonamides; and flucytosine. Trimethoprim is administered with a fixed amount of the sulfonamide sulfamethoxazole. This combination has an extended spectrum of activity which includes many aerobic Gram negative and Gram positive organisms. Ward et al found that in some cases the combination of trimethoprim-sulfamethoxazole and rifampin is effective oral treatment of methicillin resistant *Staphylococcus aureus* and *epidermidis* infections.[35] Flucytosine is an oral antifungal agent. It interferes with pyrimidine synthesis within the cell.

Pharmacokinetics of antibiotics

Successful antibiotic therapy is achieved by obtaining a concentration of antibiotic at the site of infection which is sufficient to inhibit bacterial growth and thus tips the scales in favor of the host. The concentration of the drug at the site of the infection is dependent upon the amount and frequency of drug administration and the pharmacokinetics of the drug. The pharmacokinetics of a drug encompass its absorption, distribution and elimination.

Absorption

In the management of bone and joint infections, antibiotics are most frequently given intravenously. Absorption is not an issue with intravenously administered antibiotics. Serum peak and trough concentrations are monitored and used to determine the optimum dose of toxic antibiotics which are administered intravenously. The peak serum level of an intravenously administered drug occurs shortly after administration; the trough serum level occurs immediately prior to administration.

Absorption is a factor with drugs that are administered orally and involves passage across the cell membranes of the gastrointestinal mucosa. The rate and extent of absorption of orally administered antibiotics are the key to obtaining adequate levels at the site of infection. The quinolones and metronidazole are absorbed completely from the gastrointestinal tract; vancomycin is not absorbed when given orally. Other antibiotics such as erythromycin are absorbed in varying amounts depending upon such factors as pH and concentration of calcium ions.

Distribution

To be effective the antibiotic must be distributed in such a way that therapeutic levels are reached at the site of infection. This is a troubling concept in that the site of infection is difficult to define. Technically, bacteria are in the interstitial fluid space. However, the interstitial fluid space is very different in infected bone and normal bone. In infected bone, the interstitial fluid space includes abscesses and extensive edema. We cannot assume that antibiotics will penetrate these spaces as they penetrate the interstitial fluid space of normal bone. Therefore, it is not justified to extrapolate from the normal to the diseased state. We know that antibiotics will not penetrate macroscopic areas of dead bone.[36] We do not know how large these areas must be before we see decreasing penetration. Moreover, simply studying antibiotic concentrations in various compartments may not be sufficient. Local factors such as protein binding, pH, and oxygenation affect antibiotic activity. Verwey et al have shown that protein binding decreases the activity of various antibiotics and that the concentration of binding proteins varies from compartment to compartment.[37] Verkin and Mandell, and Reynolds et al, have shown that the aminoglycosides are less active in an anaerobic, hypercapnic, acidic environment.[11,38]

With these caveats in mind, the following is known regarding antibiotic distribution. The concentration of cephalosporins, penicillin and aminoglycosides in the interstitial fluid is directly related to serum concentrations.[39,40] The penetration of penicillin and semisynthetic penicillins into synovial fluid is limited by the capillary membrane. If inflammation is present the penicillins cross the capillary membrane freely.[41]

Elimination

Antibiotics are either metabolized or excreted. Metabolism is primarily a function of the liver. Excretion is primarily a function of the kidneys. The potential for serious permanent toxicity arises when an antibiotic is toxic to the organ that is responsible for its elimination; eg, aminoglycosides are nephrotoxic and excreted by the kidney.

Therapy with antibiotic combinations

Inappropriate use of combinations of antibiotics can result in one drug inhibiting rather than enhacing the effect of the other drug. A simple rule of thumb is that bacteriostatic antibiotics frequently decrease the effectiveness of bacteriocidal drugs and that two bacteriocidal drugs may act synergistically.[42] The rationale is that bacteriostatic drugs inhibit bacterial reproduction and that the effectiveness of bactericidal drugs is dependent upon the bacteria being metabolically active and reproducing.

There are four indications for the use of combinations of antimicrobial agents. (1) The treatment of mixed bacterial infections. (2) Therapy of infections in which the specific organism is unknown. In this situation the goal of treatment is to select antibiotic coverage for all microorganisms that are most likely present. (3) The enhancement of antibacterial activity in the treatment of specific organisms. Simultaneous use of two or more antimicrobial agents frequently results in these agents acting synergistically. This synergism can be used against very resistant organisms. An example of this is the use of an aminoglycoside and a cell wall antibiotic, eg, ampicillin in the management of osteomyelitis caused by *Enterococcus*. *Enterococcus* is not sensitive to aminoglycosides because aminoglycosides do not penetrate the cell wall. However, a cell wall antibiotic increases the permeability of the cell wall to the aminoglycoside, giving it access to the interior of the cell. *Enterococcus* is extremely sensitive to this combination. Another example is the combination of one drug with another that potentiates it, eg, the beta-lactamase inhibitor clavulanic acid combined with ampicillin expands the spectrum of ampicillin to include beta-lactamase producing organisms. (4) The prevention of emergence of resistant microorganisms by mutation. The probability of independent resistance to two drugs is the product of the two frequencies of mutation which result in resistance; ie, if the frequency of mutation which results in bacterial resistance to one drug is 1 in every 10^5 cell divisions and the frequency for a second drug is 1 in every 10^{10} divisions, the probability of independent resistance to both drugs is 1 in every 10^{15} divisions. This makes the emergence of such a mutant resistance strain much less likely. This is the rationale for the use of multiple drugs in the treatment of chronic infections such as tuberculosis.

Host response to infection

Resistance to infection is divided into nonspecific and specific defenses. Nonspecific defenses include the integrity of the skin and mucous membranes, and the acute inflammatory response (eg, the undirected activity of phagocytic cells, and acute phase proteins). Specific defenses include antibody and lymphocyte mediated responses. These defenses are termed specific because they are directed at specific antigens.

Nonspecific defenses

Skin and mucous membranes

The skin presents an important mechanical barrier to bacteria. Fatty acids present on the skin and a relatively low pH inhibit bacterial replication. The outer layers of cornified epithelium are constantly shed, carrying with them bacteria which have colonized their surface. Burns, open fractures, and surgery all allow pathogenic organisms to penetrate this envelope. The respiratory tract and digestive tract also have sophisticated means of preventing bacterial penetration, including cilia, phagocytes and secretions which contain antibacterial substances.

The undirected activity of phagocytic cells

The acute inflammatory response to infection is the first response to bacterial invasion. This is an extremely complex process involving numerous cell types and humoral agents. The first cells involved are the polymorphonuclear lymphocytes (PMNs). These cells adhere to and pass through the vessel walls in the area of bacterial growth. This process of induced migration is chemotaxis. The chemotactants, or factors which cause chemotaxis, are released by the bacteria during their growth. Later in the infectious process, chemotactants are generated by the complement cascade, and by substances produced by macrophages stimulated by specific antigens. Chemotaxis is

depressed in patients with rheumatoid arthritis, correlating with a possible increased incidence of infection in these patients. The PMNs adhere to the bacteria and begin to phagocytose them. Phagocytosis is the act of a cell, when it reaches a foreign object and engulfs it, enclosing it in a cytoplasmic vacuole. This process is aided by opsonins, molecules which attach to the bacterium and make it easier to phagocytose. Opsonins are produced by the complement system and by antibodies. Following phagocytosis, cytoplasmic granules are discharged from the cell cytoplasm into the vacuole. These granules contain enzymes which kill and digest bacteria in the phagocytic vacuole. They include: phagocytin; lysozyme; cathepsin; acid phosphatase; alkaline phosphatase; nucleotidase; ribonuclease; deoxyribonuclease; and beta-glucuronidase.[43] The process of degranulation, ie, the fusion of cytoplasmic granules with the vacuoles, occurs within 30 minutes of phagocytosis.[44]

Phagocytosis and bacterial killing is not a suicidal process and the leukocytes appear to remain healthy. Exoplasmosis is the process by which phagocytic cells rid themselves of the undigested part remaining after phagocytosis. Monocytes enter the area of infection after the PMNs and eventually become the predominant cell if the infection becomes chronic or the organism is a mycobacterium or fungus. The importance of neutrophils as a host defense is illustrated by chronic granulomatous disease. This inherited disease is the result of one of four deficiencies of oxidase factors that enable leukocytes to produce oxidants. These oxidants are essential for bacterial killing. Sponseller et al reported a series of 13 patients with this disease and found that they suffered recurrent severe infections with unusual pathogens.[45]

Acute phase proteins

The third nonspecific defense against bacteria is a number of polypeptides with antibacterial activity. Because the serum concentration of these proteins changes in response to acute injury or inflammation they are called acute phase proteins.[46]

Complement system   The complement system is a series of at least 19 distinct proteins which occur in the serum and on cell membranes. Together these components account for more than 10% of serum globulins. Different elements of the complement system are produced by the liver, macrophages and intestinal mucosa. Various complement proteins combine to form complexes which activate other complement proteins. Once the complement system (or "cascade") is initiated, it proceeds to completion. The classic complement sequence is initiated by the interaction of antigen, antibody and the C1 complement protein. The complement sequence can also be initiated by the so called "alternate pathway" via tissue damage. The end result of the complement cascade is an active complex of C567 with active fragments of: C3 and C5 (these fragments are important for chemotaxis, adherence and phagocytosis); and C8 and C9 (these fragments lyse bacterial cells and also surrounding host cells). The fragments and complexes produced by the complement cascade have a direct bactericidal effect. It is termed direct because antibodies and cells are not required. Mild complement deficiencies do not increase susceptibility to infection. The complete absence of complement proteins is rare but has been reported and is associated with frequent infections, especially with Gram negative organisms.[47]

C-reactive protein   C-reactive protein was first described by Tillet and Francis in 1930.[48] Excluding the complement system it is the acute phase protein about which most is known. C-reactive protein was so named because of its calcium dependent precipitation with the C-polysaccharide of *Pneumococcus*.[46] It is a protein which is synthesized by hepatocytes, and functions primarily to enhance phagocytosis of different bacteria. In addition it is directly antibacterial as it attacks cell wall polysaccharides. C-reactive protein activates the complement system and thus enhances phagocytosis and lysis of bacteria.[49] The level of C-reactive protein in peripheral blood is used as a nonspecific indicator of infection.[50] Raised C-reactive protein levels are seen in the presence of infection, inflammation, malignancy, and tumor. After surgery the normalization time for C-reactive protein is much shorter than the erythrocyte sedimentation rate and, as such, C-reactive protein is a better indicator of postoperative infection.[51]

Interferon   This is a low molecular weight glycopeptide which is produced by infected lymphocytes. Interferon inhibits intracellular parasites, specifically DNA and RNA viruses. It does this by binding to the surface receptors of cells and by inducing enzymes that inhibit copying of viral messenger RNA into viral protein. It also increases the production of oxygen radicals by polymorphonuclear leukocytes and monocytes.[52] As such it has been administered to patients with chronic granulomatous disease.[53]

Properdin   Properdin is a beta globulin which works with the complement system and magnesium and is effective against various bacteria, viruses, protozoans, and fungi.[54]

Lysozyme   Lysozyme is a true enzyme which attacks the polymer, murein, that forms the bacterial cell wall.[55] It is effective primarily against Gram negative bacteria and also against micrococci. Lysozyme levels are low in normal patients and increased in patients with active Gram negative infections. Lysozyme also enhances the complement system.

Beta-lysins   Beta-lysins are primarily effective against Gram positive bacteria. As opposed to lysozyme, they work against the cell membrane and not the cell wall. They appear to originate from platelets.[56]

Immunoconglutinins   Immunoconglutinins are antibodies which are produced in response to antigen–complement combinations. Their lack of specificity is demonstrated by the fact that they will not bind to the antigen alone, which along with products of the complement system have stimulated their production.

Specific defenses

The immune system is termed specific because it is directed at unique individual antigens. There are two ways to look at the immune system: (1) as recognition and effector subsystems; (2) as consisting of humoral and cell mediated subsystems. Looking at the immune system as recognition and effector systems draws attention to the interdependence of the cells involved. The recognition subsystem consists of antigen recognition, processing of the antigen, and presentation of the processed antigen by the macrophages to the lymphocytes, which are then activated. The effector subsystem consists of the lymphocytes which produce antibodies (B cells), replicate to cytotoxic clones (T cells), or elaborate cytotoxins. I find it easier to understand the immune system as being divided into humoral and cell mediated arms and recognizing that these systems are interrelated. Thus, specific defenses are perceived as being either humoral or cell mediated. In this system, the result of the humoral response is antibodies, while the result of the cell mediated response is the activated T cells.

Humoral immunity

Immunoglobulins (Igs) are antibodies which interact with specific antigens and are responsible for specific humoral immunity. Igs act against bacteria by agglutinating, precipitating, immobilizing, and lysing. In addition, Igs enhance other aspects of immune function, including immune adherence, phagocytosis, and the activity of the complement system. Five different Ig classes are known. They are designated by the letters G, A, M, B, and E. IgG is the most common immunoglobulin. IgGs occur in the intravascular and extravascular spaces and have a half-life of 23 days. IgG is the most important defense against blood born pathogens, bacterial, viral, fungal, or protozoal. The second most common class of Ig is IgA. This class of Ig is found in the secretory fluids of the respiratory, genitourinary and gastrointestinal tracts. IgAs prevent colonization and infection of these surfaces by pathogenic organisms. IgMs are limited by their large size to the intravascular space. They are effective in the agglutination of particular antigens such as bacteria. IgM is the first to reach significant levels following exposure to an antigen. IgD and IgE are involved in hypersensitivity and allergic reactions. All antibodies are produced by plasma cells which are activated B lymphocytes. In man B lymphocytes originate in the liver and bone marrow. B lymphocytes have IgM and IgD molecules on their surface. Binding of an antigen to these surface receptors results in B cell proliferation, differentiation to plasma cells and antibody secretion. This process is aided by molecules (or cytokines) produced by T helper cells and macrophages.

Cell mediated immunity

Cell mediated immunity is primarily a function of T cells and is responsible for graft rejection. In bone and joint infections it is the first defense against fungal and mycotic infections and it may be an important defense in chronic bone and joint infections. T cells are produced in the bone marrow and migrate to the thymus in the fetus. Like B lymphocytes, T cells have antigen receptors on their surface. Antigen recognition by T cells requires that the antigen and a lymphokine molecule be presented together by a macrophage. Recognition of the antigen results in T cell proliferation. One of the most important lymphokines is interleukin 1 (IL1). IL1 formation is suppressed in leishmaniasis, depressing T cell function and decreasing the effectiveness of the immune system in combating this disease. T lymphocytes are directly cytotoxic by elaborating cytotoxin or indirectly by antibody dependent cytotoxicity. In addition to B and T lymphocytes there is a third type of lymphocyte, the natural killer (NK) cell. These cells are effective against tumor cells and cells infected with viruses. Macrophages and monocytes exist in an active or resting state. Resting cells have receptors for IgG, complement, and other factors on their surface. When these receptors are triggered the macrophage is activated.

References

1   Irvine GW, Kling TF, Hensinger RN, Postoperative toxic shock syndrome following osteoplasty of the hip. A case report, *J Bone Joint Surg* (1984) **66A:** 955–958.

2   Costerton JW, The etiology and persistence of cryptic bacterial infections: a hypothesis, *Rev Infect Dis* (1984) 6:608–616.

3   Gristina AG, Microbial adhesion and the pathogenesis of biomaterial-centered infections. In: Gustilo R, ed, *Orthopedic infection: diagnosis and treatment* (WB Saunders: Philadelphia 1989), 1–25.

4   Jones GW, Isaacson RE, Proteinaceous bacterial adhesions and their receptors, *Crit Rev Microbiol* (1984) **10:**229–260.

5   Speziale P, Raucci G, Visai L, et al, Binding of collagen to *Staphylococcus aureus* strain cowan I, *J Bacteriol* (1986) 167:77–81.

6   Lopes JD, dos Reis M, Brentani RR, Presence of laminin receptors in *Staphylococcus aureus*, *Science* (1985) **229:**275–277.

7   Gristina AG, Costerton JW, Bacterial adherence to biomaterials and tissue. The significance of its role in clinical sepsis, *J Bone Joint Surg* (1985) **67A:**264–273.

8   Sande MA, Mandell GL, Antimicrobial agents: general considerations. In: Goodman-Gilman A, Goodman LS, Gilman A, eds, *Goodman and Gilman's The pharmacological basis of therapeutics*, 6th edn (Macmillan: New York 1980) 1080–105.

9   Archer GL, Antimicrobial susceptibility and selection of resistance among *Staphylococcus epidermidis* isolates recovered from patients with infections of indwelling foreign devices, *Antimicrob Agents Chemother* (1978) **14:**358.

10   Strausbaugh LJ, Sande MA, L factors influencing the therapy of experimental *Proteus mirabilis* meningitis in rabbits, *J Infect Dis* (1978) 137:251–260.

11   Reynolds AV, Hamilton-Miller JM, Brumfitt W, Diminished effect of gentamicin under anaerobic and hypercapnic conditions, *Lancet* (1976) i:447.

12   Naylor PT, Myrvik QN, Gristina A, Antibiotic resistance of biomaterial-adherent coagulase-positive staphylo-cocci, *Clin Orthop Rel Res* (1990) **261:**126–133.

13   Webb LX, Gordon ES, deAraujo B, Surface adherent staphylococci and enhancement of antibiotic resistance, *Tran Ortho Res Soc* (1993) 18:455.

14   Merritt K, Boyer SA, Anderson JM, Microbial slime is a barrier to antimicrobial penetration, *Trans Ortho Res Soc* (1993) 18:457.

15   Oga M, Arizona T, Sugioka Y, Bacterial adherence to bioinert and bioactive materials studied in vitro, *Acta Orthop Scand* (1993) 63:273–276.

16 Petty W, Spanier S, Shuster JJ, et al, The influence of skeletal implants on incidence of infection. Experiments in a canine model, *J Bone Joint Surg* (1985) **67A**:1236–1244.

17 Petty W, The effect of methylmethacrylate on chemotaxis of polymorphonuclear leukocytes, *J Bone Joint Surg* (1978) **60A**:492–498.

18 Petty W, Effect of methylmethacrylate on the bacterial inhibiting properties of normal human serum, *Clin Orthop* (1978) **132**:266–278.

19 Petty W, The effect of methylmethacrylate on bacterial phagocytosis and killing by human polymorphonuclear leukocytes, *J Bone Joint Surg* (1978) **60A**:752–757.

20 Petty W, Caldwell JR, The effect of methylmethacrylate on complement activity, *Clin Orthop* (1977) **128**:354–360.

21 Gristina AG, Oga M, Webb LX, et al, Adherent bacterial colonization in the pathogenesis of osteomyelitis, *Science* (1985) **228**:990–993.

22 Marrie TJ, Costerton JW, Mode of growth of bacterial pathogens in chronic polymicrobial human osteomyelitis, *J Clin Microb* (1985) **22**:924–933.

23 Dickie P, Bryan LE, Pichard MA, Effect of enzymatic adenylation on dehydrostreptomycin accumulation in *Escherichia coli* carrying an R-factor: model explaining aminoglycoside resistance by inactivating mechanisms, *Antimicrob Agents Chemother* (1978) **14**:569–580.

24 Mandell GL, Catalase, superoxide dismutase, and virulence of *Staphylococcus aureus*, *J Clin Invest* (1975) **55**:561–566.

25 Watanabe T, Infectious drug resistance in enteric bacteria, *New Engl J Med* (1966) **275**:888–894.

26 Mader JT, Cantrell JS, Calhoun J, Oral ciprofloxacin compared with standard parenteral antibiotic therapy for chronic osteomyelitis in adults, *J Bone Joint Surg* (1990) **72A**:104–110.

27 Wilkowske CJ, Hermans PE, Actions and uses of antimicrobial agents in the treatment of musculoskeletal infections, *Orthop Clin North Am* (1975) **6**:1129–1144.

28 Sexton DJ, McDonald M, Osteomyelitis: aproaching the 1990s, *Med J Aust* (1990) **153**:91–96.

29 Kirby WM, Regamey C, Pharmacokinetics of cefazolin compared with other cephalosporins, *J Infect Dis* (1973) **128**:341.

30 Fong IW, Engelking ER, Kirby WM, Relative inactivation by *Staphylococcus aureus* of eight cephalosporin antibiotics, *Antimicrob Agents Chemother* (1076) **9**:939.

31 Kass EH, Evans DA, Future prospects and past problems in antimicrobial therapy, the role of cefoxitin, *Rev Infect Dis* (1979) **1**:1.

32 Sorrell TC, Packhan DR, Shanker S, et al, Vancomycin therapy for methicillin-resistant *Staphylococcus aureus*, *Ann Intern Med* (1982) **97**:344.

33 Veringa EM, Ferguson DA, Lambe DW, Verhoef J, The role of glycocalyx in surface phagocytosis of bacteroides spp., in the presence and abscence of clindamycin, *J Antimicrob Chemother* (1989) **23**:711–720.

34 Slama TG, Misinski J, Sklar S, Ciprofloxacin therapy of osteomyelitis, *Contemp Orthop* (1988) **16**:65–68.

35 Ward TT, Winn RE, Hartstein AI, et al, Observations relating to an inter-hospital outbreak of methicillin-resistant *Staphylococcus aureus*: role of antimicrobial therapy in

infection control, *Infect Control Hosp Epidemiol* (1981) **2**:519.

36 Perry H, Ritterbusch JK, Burdge RE, et al, Cefamandole levels in serum and necrotic bone, *Clin Orthop* (1985) **199**:280–283.

37 Verwey WF, Williams HR, Kalsow C, Penetration of chemotherapeutic agents into tissues, *Antimicrob Agents Chemother* (1965) **5**:1016–1024.

38 Verkin RM, Mandell GL, Alteration of effectiveness of antibiotics by anaerobiosis, *J Lab Clin Med* (1977) **89**:65.

39 Lunke RJ, Fitzgerald RH, Washington JA, Pharmacokinetics of cefamandole in osseous tissue, *Antimicrob Agents Chemother* (1981) **19**:851–858.

40 Fitzgerald RH, Whalen JL, Petersen SA, Pathophysiology of osteomyelitis and pharmacokinetics of antimicrobial agents in normal and osteomyelitic bone. In: Esterhai JL, Gristina AG, Poss R, eds, *Musculoskeletal infection*, 1st edn (American Academy of Orthopaedic Surgeons: Park Ridge, Illinois, 1992) 387–99.

41 Cunha BA, The use of penicillins in orthopaedic surgery, *Clin Orthop* (1984) **190**:36–50.

42 Jawetz E, Gunnison JB, Studies on antibiotic synergism and antagonism, the scheme of combined antimicrobial activity, *Antibiot Chemother* (1952) **1**:243–248.

43 Hirsch JG, Cohn ZA, Degranulation of polymorphonuclear leukocytes following phagocytosis of microorganisms, *J Exp Med* (1960) **112**:1005–1014.

44 Baggiolini M, Phagocytes use oxygen to kill bacteria, *Experimentia* (1984) **40**:906–909.

45 Sponseller PD, Malech HL, McCarthy EF, et al, Skeletal involvement in children who have chronic granulomatous disease, *J Bone Joint Surg* (1991) **73A**:37–51.

46 Carr WP, The role of laboratory in rheumatology. Acute-phase proteins, *Clin Rheuma Dis* (1983) **9**:227–239.

47 Alper CA, Propp RP, Johnston RB Jr, et al, Genetic aspects of human C'3, *J Immunol* (1968) **101**:816.

48 Tillett WS, Francis T Jr, Serological reactions in pneumonia with a non-protein somatic fraction of pneumococcus, *J Exp Med* (1930) **52**:561–571.

49 Volanakis JE, Kaplan MH, Interaction of C-reactive protein complexes with the complement system. II. Consumption of guinea-pig complement by CRP complexes: requirement for human C1q, *J Immunol* (1974) **113**:9–17.

50 Kindmark CO, Stimulating effect of C-reactive protein on phagocytosis of various species of pathogenic bacteria, *Clin Exp Immunol* (1971) **8**:941–948.

51 Larson S, Thelander U, Fribero S, C-reactive protein (CRP) levels after elective orthopedic surgery, *Clin Orthop Rel Res* (1992) **275**:237–242.

52 Nathan CF, Horowitz CR, de la Harpe J, et al, Administration of recombinant interferon gamma to cancer patients enhances monocyte secretion of hydrogen peroxide, *Proc Nat Acad Sci* **82**:8686–8690, 1985.

53 Heinrich SD, Finney T, Craver R, et al, Aspergillus osteomyelitis in patients who have chronic granulomatous disease. A case report, *J Bone Joint Surg* (1991) **73A**:456–460.

54 Wardlaw AC, Pillemer L, The properdin system and immunity. The bactericidal activity

of the properdin system, *J Exp Med* (1956) **103**:553–573.

55   Mandelstam J, Isolation of lysozyme-soluble mucopeptides from the cells wall of *Escherichia coli*, *Nature* (1961) **189**:855–856.

56   Matheson A, Donaldson DM, Alterations in the morphology of *Bacillus subtilis* after exposure to B-lysin and ultraviolet light, *J Bacteriol* (1968) **95**:1892–1902.

3
CLASSIFICATION AND PATHOPHYSIOLOGY

Bone and joint infections fall into one of five basic groups: osteomyelitis (acute or chronic); infections of the spine; infections of the lower extremity in the diabetic; septic arthritis; and septic arthroplasties. These are distinct entities and are discussed separately.

Acute and chronic osteomyelitis

Osteomyelitis literally means inflammation of bone and marrow elements. We use the term osteomyelitis to denote bacterial or, occasionally, fungal infections of bone. The bacteria reach the bone hematogenously (ie, by embolizing through the circulatory system) or via direct inoculation. Direct inoculation occurs when bacteria spread from a contiguous focus of infection (eg, a mal-perforans ulcer) or by surgical or traumatic introduction of bacteria to the bone (eg, an open tibia fracture). Peripheral vascular disease has been cited as a third cause of osteomyelitis. However, it is clear that while dysvascularity may increase the susceptibility to osteomyelitis, it is not the actual cause of infection.[1]

Osteomyelitis is acute or chronic. We arbitrarily define osteomyelitis as being acute if it has been symptomatic less than four weeks. After four weeks of symptoms we define it as chronic. A less arbitrary and more accurate definition is that osteomyelitis is acute as long as the predominant histologic and clinical picture is that of acute infection. When chronic inflammation and the secondary changes due to dysvascularity and scarring begin, the disease is defined as chronic. Even this definition is unclear because chronic osteomyelitis is frequently complicated by acute flare-ups.

Acute osteomyelitis

Clinically, the diagnosis of acute osteomyelitis is based on the presence of pain and swelling. Frequently the patient will be systemically ill. When the infection is hematogenous in origin, the patient is usually skeletally immature and the metaphysis of a long bone is involved. When the infection is secondary to direct inoculation, there is a history of a break in the skin due to an injury, surgery, or an ulcer. The definitive diagnosis of osteomyelitis is made by growing organisms in culture from pus or tissue obtained from around the questionable area.

Acute hematogenous osteomyelitis

Acute hematogenous osteomyelitis is primarily a disease of growing bone and affects males twice as frequently as females. The infection invariably starts in the metaphysis. There are two theories as to why this is so. The most reasonable is based on Trueta and Morgan's observation that the capillary ramifications of the nutrient artery turn away from the growth plate and empty into much larger sinusoidal veins.[2,3] (Fig. 3.1). These afferent capillaries are "end vessels", and obstruction secondary to thrombus or bacterial growth results in microscopic areas of avascular

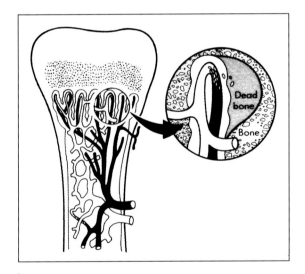

Figure 3.1

Hematogenous osteomyelitis starts in the metaphysis where the capillaries turn away from the physis and empty into larger vinous sinusoids. In this area of slow blood flow, blood born bacteria adhere to the bone through endothelial gaps. The bacteria reproduce and the vessel thromboses.

necrosis. Therefore, in the area of the metaphysis adjacent to the physis, there is decreased oxygen tension, slow, turbulent blood flow and the blood supply is precarious. The low oxygen tension decreases the phagocytic activity of granulocytes and macrophages.[2,4,5] The turbulent flow allows bacteria to adhere to the exposed matrix adjacent to the endothelial gaps in the growing metaphyseal vessels. When end vessels thrombose, avascular areas of bone result, decreasing the effectiveness of host defenses. In addition, Hobo felt that there is a paucity of macrophages in the proximal metaphysis, further increasing the susceptibility to infection.[5] Emslie and Nade developed an avian model in which staphylococcal osteomyelitis was induced by injection of bacteria.[6,7] Their model provides tangible evidence that confirms Trueta and Morgan's theory of pathogenesis.[2,3] Morrissy et al and then Whalen et al disputed this theory and offered an alternative hypothesis.[8,9] These investigators found no anatomic connection between the capillaries and the efferent venules. They felt that microscopic trauma to the physis lowered resistance to infection. And they were able to produce osteomyelitis in rabbits by fracturing the metaphysis and then inoculating the animal with bacteria. They do not suggest where the afferent capillaries drain or what the function of the venules is. Nor do they explain why children who have had radiographically obvious fractures of the metaphysis and physis rarely develop a hematogenous infection.

Regardless of whether the infection starts in the metaphysis because of the idiosyncrasies of the circulation of growing long bones or because of microtrauma, the fact is that almost all hematogenous infections originate in the metaphysis.[10,11] As the bacteria reproduce and their number increases the host responds. This acute inflammatory response by the host either eradicates the bacteria or results in an abscess. If an abscess results, it expands by moving along the lines of least resistance and fills the medullary canal (Fig. 3.2). The nutrient artery of the bone involved frequently thromboses. At the same

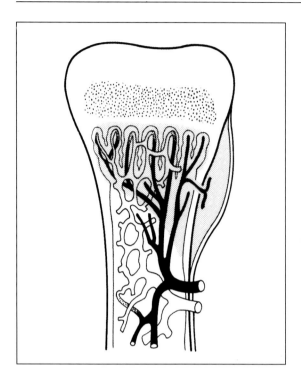

Figure 3.2

An intramedullary abscess develops and travels along vascular channels, through the cortex, where it lifts the periosteum and forms a subperiosteal abscess.

time, contents of the abscess migrate via the Haversian systems, Volkmann's canals and along thrombosed nutrient arteries through the cortex and collect under the periosteum. There they form the classic metaphyseal subperiosteal abscess. As the periosteum is elevated from the underlying bone by the subperiosteal abscess, the bone becomes avascular, forming a sequestrum. The periosteum continues to lay down bone, but at a distance from the original bone. This new bone is termed an involucrum. Infection rarely extends to the epiphysis because the physis serves as a barrier to infection. The two important exceptions to this rule are infants and adults. Infants up to six months of age have capillaries which traverse the physis. Bacteria often spread via these capillaries to the epiphysis and then intraarticularly, destroying the epiphysis and causing joint sepsis. In adults the physis has been resorbed and therefore it no longer serves as a barrier.[2]

At the point that a subperiosteal abscess is formed the histologic findings have been grouped into three characteristic zones. There is a central zone of necrotic tissue, fibrin deposits, and polymorphonuclear leukocytes. The central zone is surrounded by a zone of granulation tissue, lymphocytes and plasma cells. The third, outer zone consists of fibrous tissue and new bone. The prominence of a zone determines the histologic and to a large degree clinical appearance of the disease.[12] For example, in acute pyogenic osteomyelitis the predominant histologic picture is that of the central zone: necrotic tissue, fibrin, and polymorphonuclear leukocytes. Clinically, the patient is ill and has the signs and symptoms of an acute infection. As acute osteomyelitis becomes chronic, histologic findings compatible with the outer two zones begin to predominate. Lymphocytes, plasma cells, granulation tissue and new bone begin to appear. In Brodie's abscess, or subacute pyogenic osteomyelitis, there is almost no purulent material but rather a cavity of granulation tissue surrounded by fibrous tissue and sclerotic bone. Clinically, the patient is not systemically ill but does have symptoms compatible with a localized infection. In sclerosing osteomyelitis of Garré the outer zone predominates to the exclusion of the inner two zones. There is no purulent material and minimal granulation tissue but marked fibrosis and periosteal bone formation. Although this condition may involve any bone it most commonly affects the mandible and is caused by *Staphylococcus aureus*.[12]

Direct inoculation

Acute osteomyelitis secondary to direct inoculation occurs in three distinct clinical situations: following trauma; following surgery; and by spread from a contiguous focus. All three of these situations share an underlying cause, ie, a break in the skin that allows the ingress of bacteria. In addition there is an area of damaged bone or soft tissue surrounding the bone in which bacteria can grow. When bacteria are introduced into this environment their initial growth stimulates an acute inflammatory response by the host. If the bacteria are not eradicated, acute osteomyelitis, as indicated by abscess formation, pain, erythema and swelling, results. Abscesses will expand along the lines of least resistance, and usually spontaneously drain to the outside; however, they may expand along compromised tissue planes.

Predisposing factors

The pathogenic organism must be definitively determined from culture of material obtained by aspiration or biopsy. However, between the time that the diagnosis of osteomyelitis is made and the results of the cultures are available, antibiotics are initiated. The antibiotics are selected based upon the factors which predispose patients to specific organisms, so that appropriate antibiotic therapy can be initiated (Table 3.1). Gram negative rods and group B streptococci are important pathogens in neonates; in older children *Staphylococcus aureus* is the most frequent pathogen. In patients with sickle cell disease *Staphylococcus* and *Salmonella* cause hematogenous osteomyelitis. There is some controversy as to which organism is the most common pathogen. Epps et al found almost equal numbers of patients with staphylococcal and *Salmonella* osteomyelitis.[13] Vichinsky and Lubin reported a low incidence of *Salmonella* osteomyelitis in patients with sickle cell hemoglobinopathy, while Mallouh and Talab reported an incidence of 85%.[14,15] Mallouh and Talab attribute this disparity to the "high prevalence of infection with *Salmonella* in this part of the world [Saudi Arabia]".[15] The pathogenesis of *Salmonella* osteomyelitis is that small infarcts in the intestinal wall lead to periodic hematogenous showers of intestinal flora. If *Salmonella* is not usually part of this flora (as is the case in the United States), the incidence of *Salmonella* osteomyelitis will be correspondingly low.

Table 3.1   Common predisposing factors and corresponding pathogens leading to osteomyelitis

Predisposing factors	Pathogens
Infancy	Group B streptococci
Childhood	*Haemophilus influenzae*
Sickle cell disease	*Salmonella* sp.
Immunosuppression	Opportunistic fungi, *Nocardia*, *Pseudomonas*
Residing in an endemic area	*Coccidiodes immitis*, *Histoplasma capsulatum*
Trauma to the jaw	*Actinomyces israelii*
Animal exposure	*Brucella* sp.
Pulmonary tuberculosis	*Mycobacterium tuberculosis*

Chronic osteomyelitis

The diagnosis of chronic osteomyelitis is based on the presence of chronic drainage from sinuses, fistulas, or ulcers. There is almost always a history of acute osteomyelitis. An acute "flare-up", as indicated by pain and swelling, may be superimposed on chronic osteomyelitis. The patient is seldom systemically ill, in contrast to patients with acute osteomyelitis. The diagnosis is confirmed by growing organisms in culture from material obtained from the area in question.

Cierny et al classified adult chronic osteomyelitis into 12 groups[16] (Table 3.2). These groups have implications regarding management and prognosis. They do not necessarily have implications regarding the origin or pathophysiology of the infection. This classification system is based upon the location and extent of involvement of the bone and the physiologic status of the patient. Location and extent of involvement is classified into four groups (Fig. 3.3): superficial, in which only the outer surface of the cortex is involved; medullary, in which the medullary canal is involved; localized, in which a full thickness area of cortex is involved; and diffuse, in which there is segmental involvement. The physiologic status of the patient is classified into three groups: an A host is a patient who can mount a normal response to infection; a B host is one who cannot mount a normal response to infection because of either local compromise (eg, a dysvascular extremity) or systemic compromise (eg, malnutrition); a C host is a patient for whom treatment is worse than the effects of the disease. This is usually because the disease is minimally symptomatic or the required therapy is so extensive that its risk outweighs that of the infection. The management implications of this classification system are that: more extensive involvement requires more extensive resection and reconstruction; B hosts should be changed to A hosts prior to therapy; and C hosts should not be treated. The prognostic implications of this classification system are that more extensive involvement and compromise of the host carry a poor prognosis.

May et al have classified posttraumatic osteomyelitis of the tibia[17] (Fig. 3.4). Their classification is based upon the status of the tibia. Type I is an intact tibia and fibula capable of withstanding functional loads. Type II is an intact tibia with

Table 3.2   Classification of chronic osteomyelitis

Location and extent of infection	Physiologic status		
	A	B	C
1	1A	1B	1C
2	2A	2B	2C
3	3A	3B	3C
4	4A	4B	4C

Location and extent of infection: type 1, superficial; type 2, medullary; type 3, localized; type 4, diffuse.
Physiologic status: group A, normal; group B, compromised; group C, treatment worse than disease.
Example: 4B is a diffuse osteomyelitis in a compromised patient.

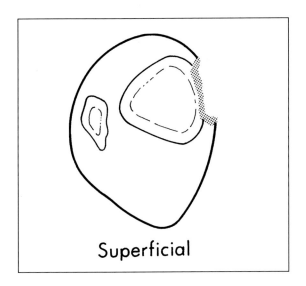

Figure 3.3a

Superficial osteomyelitis involves only part of the cortex. A full thickness skin burn might precede this type of osteomyelitis.

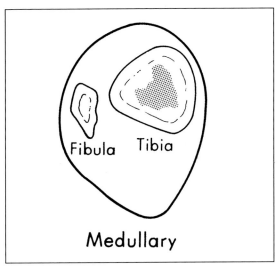

Figure 3.3b

Medullary osteomyelitis is limited to the medullary canal. The cortex is not involved. Medullary osteomyelitis is often a complication of intramedullary nailing.

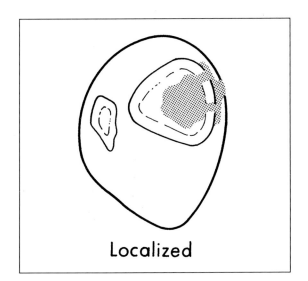

Figure 3.3c

Localized osteomyelitis involves the entire thickness of the cortex, and is often caused by application of a plate.

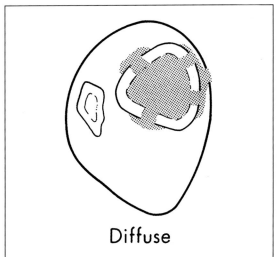

Figure 3.3d

Diffuse osteomyelitis involves a segment of bone. It represents superficial, medullary, or localized osteomyelitis which has been allowed to progress, or an infected nonunion.

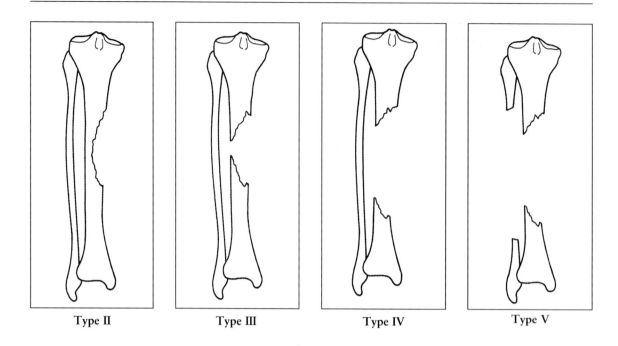

| Type II | Type III | Type IV | Type V |

Figure 3.4

May's classification system of osteomyelitis of the tibia. Type I is not shown.

bone graft needed for structural support. Type III is a tibial defect 6 cm long or less and intact fibula. Type IV is a tibial defect more than 6 cm long and intact fibula. .Type V is a tibial defect more than 6 cm long and no usable intact fibula. This classification system is designed to direct bony reconstruction of the débrided tibia. However, it is of limited use because: it does not include some of the most commonly encountered situations (eg, a hypertrophic or atrophic non-union with a fibula which is not intact); it does not take into account malunion or the condition of the soft tissue (eg, nerves, arteries, veins, skin, and muscle); or the age and demands of the patient and the presence of diseases such as diabetes.[18]

Infections of the spine

Infections of the spine involve the vertebral bodies, the intervertebral discs, or both. Spine infections differ from other bone and joint infections regarding: pathogenesis; clinical and laboratory findings; and complications.

Pathogenesis of hematogenous spine infections

This discussion does not pertain to postoperative wound infections of the spine. In the adult, hematogenous infections of the spine most commonly start in the vertebral body and spreads to the disc space secondarily. Batson suggested that hematogenous spread of prostatic metastasis to the vertebrae was via the pelvic venous plexus (Batson's plexus).[19] Wiley and Trueta found that the venous system drained the bladder and surrounding area and could be filled retrograde if positive pressure was applied, inferring that not only metastasis but also bacteria could spread to the vertebrae via Batson's plexus.[20] That bacteria seed the vertebral bodies via Batson's plexus is supported by a study reported by Digby and Kersley.[21] They found that pyogenic osteomyelitis followed urinary tract instrumentation in 13 of the 30 cases studied. However, the fact that endplates of two adjoining vertebrae occasionally appear to be involved simultaneously suggests that in these cases bacterial seeding may be via arteries. Once in the adult vertebra, the bacteria lodge in the low flow vascular arcades adjacent to the vertebral endplates. The leukocyte response to the proliferation of these bacteria results in local destruction of bony trabecula and erosion of the endplates overlying the avascular disc. Bacteria and the products of inflammation can then involve the disc. The disc herniates through the endplate into the vertebral body. At the same time the nucleus pulposus involutes because of loss of water from its substance. Disc herniation and involution of the nucleus pulposus result in narrowing of the disc space, often the first tangible radiographic sign of infection. The inevitable disc space narrowing has led to the erroneous term "disc space infection" when referring to adult vertebral osteomyelitis.

Vertebral osteomyelitis of adults is distinct from disc space infection, or discitis, of children. Coventry et al showed that in children there are vascular channels perforating the vertebral endplates which provide a pathway for hematogenous spread of bacteria to the disc itself.[22] These vascular channels disappear by the age of 30 years. While most investigators believe that the infection starts in the disc in children, some

believe that it starts near the vertebral endplate of the vertebral body, much the same as in adults.[23]

Clinical and laboratory findings of spine infections

Usually the age of onset of vertebral osteomyelitis is after 40 years of age. Urinary tract infections, intravenous drug abuse, and diabetes are risk factors. The primary symptom is back pain, the onset of which is usually insidious and progressive. As in other infections this pain is not relieved by rest or analgesics. The most constant physical finding is pain to palpation at the level of involvement. The leukocyte count may be normal, although the erythrocyte sedimentation rate is usually elevated. T-11 to L-4 are involved most frequently. Pathogenic organisms are most frequently *Staphylococcus aureus* or Gram negative organisms, the latter being found more frequently in intravenous drug abusers. There is a greater incidence of fungal and mycobacterial pathogens in the spine than elsewhere.

The clinical findings of disc space infection in children are similar to those of vertebral osteomyelitis in adults. Boston et al found that the predominant symptom was pain; in addition they found that 10 of 19 children with spine infections had a significant elevation in their temperature.[24] Wenger et al found that while the predominant symptom was pain, in 6 of the 41 patients in their study the pain was localized to the abdomen and not the back.[23] Cultures of material obtained from disc biopsy and blood cultures are negative in about 50% of children with discitis, indicating a possible viral etiology in the 50% who are culture negative. When cultures are positive, *Staphylococcus aureus* is usually the pathogenic organism. As in adults with vertebral osteomyelitis, the radiographic hallmark of discitis is collapse of the disc space due to decreased water binding capacity of the nucleus pulposus and herniation of disc material into the vertebral bodies. Eradication of symptoms is invariably accomplished with bedrest only, although usually antibiotics are also administered.[24]

Tuberculous osteomyelitis of the spine is rare in developed countries, but should be included in the differential diagnosis of any patient with an infected spine. The most important risk factor is an already existing active focus of tubercular infection (eg, an infected hip). The level of involvement is similar to that of pyogenic vertebral osteomyelitis, and is most frequently between the T-10 and L-4 vertebrae. Radiographically there are frequently large paravertebral abscesses, and involvement of the posterior elements. Other radiographic signs indicating mycobacterial osteomyelitis as opposed to pyogenic osteomyelitis are: "concertina collapse" of a vertebrae, when the entire vertebra, weakened by the ingrowth of granulation tissue, collapses radially, often resulting in neurologic compromise; aneurysmal syndrome, due to a long paravertebral abscess; wedging of the spine due to partial collapse of a vertebra (Pott's disease if it results in kyphosis, but lateral wedging also occurs); and calcification of the intervertebral discs.[25]

Complications of spine infections

The complication unique to vertebral osteomyelitis is paralysis. Eismont et al, in a study of 61 patients with pyogenic or fungal vertebral osteomyelitis, identified the following risk factors: age – no patient under the age of 37 years developed paralysis; location – patients with cervical involvement had the highest incidence of paralysis, those with lumbar involvement the lowest incidence; rheumatoid arthritis, diabetes, and steroids – all patients with rheumatoid arthritis, 10 of 12 patients with diabetes, and 5 of 6 patients taking steroids developed paralysis; and *Staphylococcus aureus* as the pathogen – 7

of 8 patients with the "most severe" paralysis were infected with *Staphylococcus aureus*. Eismont et al stress the necessity of decompressing vertebral osteomyelitis anteriorly, as the posterior elements are uninvolved and are stabilizing the spinal column.[26] They found that half of the patients who underwent anterior decompression improved or remained unchanged, whereas the patients who underwent posterior decompression worsened or remained unchanged.

Infected lower extremity in the diabetic

The foot of the diabetic is particularly susceptible to infection. When infection occurs it is classified into one of six grades: 0, skin intact (may have bony deformity); 1, localized superficial ulcer; 2, deep ulcer to tendon or bone; 3, deep abscess or osteomyelitis; 4, necrosis of toes or forefoot; and 5, necrosis of entire foot. The increased susceptibility to infection of the diabetic foot is due to angiopathy, neuropathy, and immunopathy.[27]

Angiopathy

Diabetics have two types of vascular lesions: the macrolesion, or atherosclerotic lesion; and the microlesion. Macrolesions also occur in nondiabetics, but in diabetics: they occur at a younger age and are more severe; they are more diffuse, with multisegment involvement; vessels distal to the trifurcation are more frequently involved; and both lower extremities are more frequently involved. Microlesions also occur in the nondiabetic as part of the normal aging process. These lesions consist of thickening of the capillary basement membrane, and they are more extensive in insulin dependent diabetics. This thickening of the basement membrane is a generalized process found in many types of tissue. Thus, both types of vascular lesions occur in nondiabetics, but in diabetics they occur at an earlier age, at a greater frequency and progress more rapidly to a more advanced stage.[28]

Neuropathy

Diabetic neuropathy is typically distal and symmetric, ie, stocking distribution. Theories of the cause of the neuropathy include: basement membrane thickening of the Schwann cell sheaths; metabolic disturbances of nerve cells; and decreased axonal transport.[29] The first signs of neuropathy are usually paresthesias, followed by loss of proprioception hypesthesia, muscle wasting and loss of reflexes. The combination of angiopathy and neuropathy results in a number of poorly understood problems, including neuropathic joints, nail enlargement, and callous hypertrophy.

Immunopathy

The immunopathy of the diabetic appears to be at the cellular level, specifically: decreased chemotaxis of polymorphonuclear leukocytes; impaired intracellular killing, and impaired lymphocyte transformation. Both of these defects are made worse by hyperglycemia.[30–33]

Acute and chronic septic arthritis

Septic arthritis is a relatively common occurrence with a confusingly large number of etiologies. The diagnosis of septic arthritis is usually obvious. The physical signs are a swollen, hot, painful joint. The patient will frequently be systemically ill. The affected joint is held motionless in the position in which there is maximum room in the capsule, ie, the knee at 30°, the hip flexed

and externally rotated. Any attempt to move the joint results in severe pain. Polymorphonuclear leukocytes and bacteria obtained on aspiration of the joint give the definitive diagnosis. The differential diagnosis includes aseptic arthritis due to crystals (eg, gout and pseudogout) or autoimmune disease.

There are three parameters by which septic arthritis is classified: the mode of entry of the pathogenic organisms into the joint; the chronicity of infection; and the identity of the pathogenic organisms.

Mode of entry

Pathogenic bacteria gain entrance to a joint by one of three routes: hematogenously; direct inoculation; and contiguous spread.

Hematogenous

The most frequent mode of ingress is hematogenous spread. The incidence of hematogenous infections is biphasic, being more common in infants and the skeletally mature than it is in children.[34] This is because in childhood the avascular physeal plate serves as a barrier to the spread of infection from the metaphysis (see page 28), whereas in infants vessels penetrate the physis and in adults the physis has been resorbed. The incidence of hematogenous septic arthritis is the same in males and females, as opposed to hematogenous osteomyelitis in which males are involved twice as frequently. The hip is the joint most commonly involved in infants, the knee in children and adults. Hematogenous septic arthritis of the shoulder has a particularly bad prognosis. Leslie et al reported a series of 18 patients with infected shoulders.[35] Two patients died, and the remaining 16 patients had a poor functional result. These poor results are explained by the fact that there was a delay in diagnoses in 17 patients,

17 patients had at least one serious systemic disease, and the age of the patients ranged from 42 to 80 years. My experience with septic shoulders has been similar, in that the patients seem to be older, and more debilitated, than patients with septic knees and hips.

Direct inoculation

When septic arthritis is secondary to direct inoculation of the joint with bacteria, there is a history of surgery (e.g., arthroscopy) or trauma (e.g., laceration of the metacarpal phalangeal joint). Infection following arthroscopy is rare. Sherman et al reviewed 2640 arthroscopies of the knee.[36] Infection was defined as when purulent fluid was aspirated from the knee and at least one organism was isolated. They found that the rate of infection was less than 0.2%,

and that it was approximately three times less following diagnostic arthroscopy than when an intraarticular procedure was performed. This low incidence of infection can prevent adequate management in that the surgeon will ignore symptoms indicative of joint sepsis, or manage them empirically with oral antibiotics. Laceration of the metacarpal phalangeal joint is usually sustained in a fight when the clenched fist strikes a sharp object, eg a tooth (Figs 3.5 and 3.6). The laceration extends through the skin, extensor hood, and joint capsule. Frequently the metacarpal head has a small impaction fracture. The tooth carries pathogenic organisms that seed the joint. When the hand is held in the position of rest with the metacarpal phalangeal joint flexed 30°, the extensor hood is pulled proximally, sealing closed the laceration in the capsule. As the pathogenic organisms in the joint begin to reproduce the signs and symptoms of an abscess develop (see Figs 3.5 and 3.6).

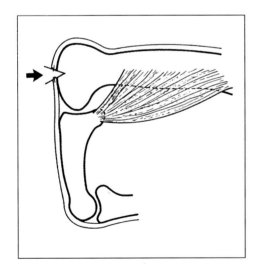

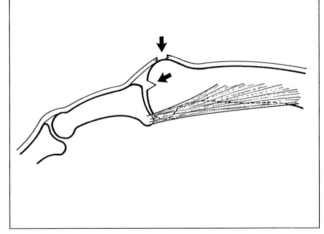

Figure 3.5

When the clenched fist strikes a sharp object, the skin and extensor hood is lacerated, and bacteria may be carried into the metacarpal phalangeal joint.

Figure 3.6

When the hand is held in the position of rest, the joint is sealed, preventing drainage, and facilitating bacterial reproduction.

Spread from contiguous focus

The third route by which pathogenic bacteria gain entrance to a joint is via a contiguous focus of infection. This is most frequently metaphyseal osteomyelitis that drains into a joint. Although this mode of ingress can occur with virtually any joint, those joints in which the metaphysis is intracapsular are at greater risk, in particular the hip, shoulder, and elbow. The clinical significance of this is that when septic arthritis is diagnosed, metaphyseal osteomyelitis must be ruled out.

Chronicity of infection

Regardless of the mode of entry of bacteria or the identity of the bacteria, septic arthritis is described as being in the acute, subacute, or chronic stage. In the acute stage the host responds to intraarticular bacteria by synovial proliferation and exudation of fluid, which causes joint distention. Polymorphonuclear leukocytes enter the joint capsule and, in the process of phagocytosing bacteria, empty their proteolytic enzymes into the synovial fluid. It is these enzymes that begin the destruction of the hyaline cartilage lining of the joint surfaces and the cruciate ligaments. When irreversible damage to these intraarticular structures has occurred the process is in the subacute stage. As the subacute stage continues, a pannus of synovial tissue grows over the intraarticular structures. This synovial tissue elaborates lytic enzymes which erode underlying structures, including articular cartilage. The containment of large volumes of purulent material within the joint capsule distends the joint, resulting in laxity and eventually subluxation. When damage to extraarticular structures has occurred, the infection is in the chronic stage. Chronic septic joints have one or more of the following: destruction of the joint; osteomyelitis; joint subluxation or dislocation; ankylosis; fracture; and avascular necrosis.

Pathogenic organism

Septic arthritis is also classified according to the pathogenic organisms into five groups: Gram positive aerobes and *Haemophilus*; Gram negative aerobes; anaerobes; mycobacteria and fungi; gonococci and Lyme disease. This classification directs the management of acute and chronic infections and is covered in Chapter 7. The relative incidence of specific pathogens is illustrated in Table 3.3.

Lyme disease is a relatively recently recognized entity which can result in septic arthritis. It is caused by the spirochete *Borrelia burgdorferi*, is transmitted through the bite of the deer tick, *Ixodes dammini*, and is limited primarily to the northern half of the United States. Lyme disease involves multiple systems, including the nervous system, heart, and the skin. The disease has three stages. Stage 1 occurs within 30 days of the bite of the deer tick and consists of erythema migrans, or an expanding red ring around the bite. Stage 2 occurs 14 days to several months after the bite. It consists of cardiac (arrhythmias) and neurologic manifestations (Bell's palsy) of the disease. Less than 20% of infected patients develop symptoms indicative of stage 2. Stage 3 is the arthritic stage of the disease. The knee is the most frequently involved joint, with the hip, ankle, shoulder, and elbow also frequently involved. Arthritis can be migratory, explaining why Lyme disease was mistaken for juvenile rheumatoid arthritis until recently. Although autoimmune complexes are found in the synovial fluid, this is not just an autoimmune complex. Spirochetes have been isolated from the synovial tissue of involved joints and high dose penicillin therapy usually results in cure.[37,38]

Table 3.3   Most frequent causes of bacterial arthritis by age

Organism	0–2 months	2 months to 2 years	3–10 years	11 years and over
Staphylococcus aureus	25%	10%	25%	50%
Streptococcus species (group A, pneumoniae)	10%	10%	25%	10%
Group B streptococci	25%	Rare	Rare	10%
Haemophilus influenzae	Rare	50%	10%	Rare
Neisseria	Rare	10%	25%	10%[a]
Gram negative bacilli	25%	10%	10%	10%
Anaerobes	Rare	Rare	Rare	Rare

[a] Generally adults less than 30 years of age.

Septic arthroplasties

Pathogenesis

Infection following a total joint arthroplasty is either due to inoculation of the joint with bacteria in the perioperative period (ie, at the time of surgery or in the immediate postoperative period) or is via hematogenous spread at some time after the postoperative period. The number and types of pathogenic organisms are similar in postoperative, or early, and hematogenous, or late prosthetic infections. This raises the possibility that many so called hematogenous prosthetic infections may in fact be postoperative infections that have remained dormant after surgery. Clearly, there are cases of hematogenous infection following dental manipulation, in which the pathogenic organism is normal oral flora. For example, Strazzeri and Anzel reported a case of *Actinomyces israelii* infecting a total hip arthroplasty after dental extraction, and Sullivan et al reported a case of *Peptostreptococcus* infecting a total hip arthroplasty after repair of a dental crown.[39,40] Whether the infection is postsurgical or hematogenous in origin, bacteria adhere to the surface of the prosthesis either in the joint itself or at the bone prosthesis interface. Here they are in a protected environment. As they reproduce, the host response results in either a septic joint or an abscess at the bone–prosthesis interface.

Incidence

The incidence of postsurgical infection following a total joint arthroplasty is 1–2%. The incidence of hematogenous infection is difficult to determine but is probably less than 1%. Certain risk factors have been identified. Poss et al studied 4240 hip, knee and elbow arthroplasties.[41] They found that: patients with rheumatoid arthritis had a 2.6 times greater risk than patients with osteoarthritis; patients undergoing a revision hip arthroplasty had an 8 times greater risk than patients undergoing a primary arthroplasty; patients with metal to metal hinged knee prosthesis were 20 times more likely to become infected than patients with metal to plastic prosthesis; and that patients with total elbow arthroplasties were 10 times more likely to become infected than patients with total hip or knee arthroplasties. Murray et al reported a series of 68 patients who had undergone two or more arthroplasties of major joints, one of which had become infected.[42] Ten of these 68 patients subsequently developed an infection of the second arthroplasty, indicating that a previously infected arthroplasty is a significant risk factor for infection of a second arthroplasty.

Clinical laboratory and radiographic findings

The rate of onset of infection and clinical picture is dependent somewhat upon the pathogenic organism and the ability of the patient to mount a host response. Beta-hemolytic *Streptococcus* and *Staphylococcus aureus* may cause a fulminant infection and the patient will present in septic shock. More frequently, the physical findings of an acute septic arthroplasty are pain and swelling. The pain is characteristic in that it is unremitting and is not relieved by rest or physical therapy. If the infection is postsurgical, there is usually drainage through the wound. Hematogenous infections may have been preceded by genitourinary or dental manipulation. Frequently the patient has had flu-like symptoms for several days preceding the joint symptoms. The diagnosis is confirmed by growing organisms in culture from material obtained from the joint. The incidence of specific pathogens causing total joint infections varies from that causing osteomyelitis. In general *Staphylococcus epidermidis* and *Streptococcus* are more common causes of infection in total joint arthroplasties. In a report of 63 infected knee and hip prostheses, Inman et al found that the pathogenic organism was *Staphylococcus epidermidis* in 25% of cases, *Staphylococcus aureus* in 12% of cases, and *Streptococcus* group A, B, or *faecalis* in 12% of cases.[43]

Radiographically the signs of bone–prosthesis interface involvement are focal osteolysis followed by a radiolucent zone around the prosthesis and eventual loosening. The differentiation of septic arthritis from bone–prosthesis interface involvement is potentially important as a septic arthritis can theoretically be managed with local antibiotics and leaving the prosthesis *in situ*. In addition, infection of the bone–prosthesis interface may carry a worse prognosis than a septic arthritis as antibiotics, polymorphonuclear leukocytes, and serum antibacterial factors may not penetrate this interface. This is particularly true if PMMA has been used because the heat of polymerization kills the endosteal bone and destroys the circulation adjacent to the interface. Involvement of the bone–prosthesis interface mandates removal of the prosthesis to clear the infection.

References

1   Waldvogel FA, Medoff G, Swartz MN, Osteomyelitis: a review of clinical features, therapeutic considerations and unusual aspects (first of three parts), *New Engl J Med* (1970) **282**:198–320.

2   Trueta J, The three types of acute hematogenous osteomyelitis, a clinical and vascular study, *J Bone Joint Surg* (1959) **41B**:671–680.

3   Morgan JD, Blood supply of growing rabbit's tibia, *J Bone Joint Surg* (1959) **41B**:185–203.

4   Moelleken BRW, Mathes SJ, Hunt TK, A poorly vascularized wound adversely affects neutrophil function. In: Esterhai JL, Gristina AG, Poss R, eds, *Musculoskeletal infection*, 1st edn (American Academy of Orthopaedic Surgeons: Park Ridge, Illinois, 1992) 367–86.

5 Hobo T, Zur pathogenese der akuten haematogenen Osteomyelitis, *Acta Med Univ Kiota* (1921) **4**:1–29.

6 Emslie KR, Nade S, Acute hematogenous staphylococcal osteomyelitis. A description of the natural history in an avian model, *Am J Pathol* (1983) **110**:333–345.

7 Norden CW, Lessons learned from animal models of osteomyelitis, *Rev Infect Dis* (1988) **10**:103–110.

8 Morrissy RT, Haynes DW, Nelson CL, Acute hematogenous osteomyelitis: the role of trauma in a reproducible model, *Trans Orthop Res Soc* (1980) **5**:324.

9 Whalen JL, Fitzgerald RH, Morrissy RT, A histological study of acute hematogenous osteomyelitis following physeal injuries in rabbits, *J Bone Joint Surg* (1988) **70A**:1382–1392.

10 Green NE, Edwards K, Bone and joint infections in children, *Orthop Clin North Am* (1987) **18**:555–576.

11 Hoyt WA, Davis AE, Van Buren G, Acute hematogenous staphylococcic osteomyelitis, *JAMA* (1941) **117**:2043–2050.

12 Lennert K, Grundprobleme der osteomyelitis, *Verh Deutsch Orthop Ges* (1963) **51**:27–64.

13 Epps CH, Bryant DD, Coles MJ, et al, Osteomyelitis in patients who have sickle cell disease. Diagnosis and management, *J Bone Joint Surg*, (1991) **73A**:1281–1294.

14 Vichinsky EP, Lubin BH, Sickle cell anemia and related hemoglobinopathies, *Ped Clin North Am* (1980) **27**:429–447 .

15 Mallouh A, Talab Y, Bone and joint infections in patients with sickle cell disease, *J Ped Orthop* (1985) **5**:158–162.

16 Cierny G, Mader JT, Penninck JJ, A clinical staging system for adult osteomyelitis, *Contemp Orthop* (1985) **10**:17–37.

17 May JW, Jupiter JB, Weland AJ, et al, Current concepts review, clinical classification of post-traumatic osteomyelitis, *J Bone Joint Surg* (1989) **71A**:1422–1428.

18 Stauffer RN, Pyogenic vertebral osteomyelitis, *Orthop Clin North Am* (1975) **6**:1015–1027.

19 Batson OV, The function of the vertebral veins and their role in the spread of metastases, *Ann Surg* (1940) **112**: 138–149.

20 Wiley AM, Trueta J, The vascular anatomy of the spine and its relationship to pyogenic vertebral osteomyelitis, *J Bone Joint Surg* (1959) **41B**:796–809.

21 Digby JM, Kersley JB, Pyogenic non-tuberculous spinal infection, an analysis of thirty cases, *J Bone Joint Surg* (1979) **61B**:47–55.

22 Coventry MB, Ghormley RK, Kernohan JW, The intervertebral disc: its microscopic anatomy and pathology, *J Bone Joint Surg* (1945) **27**:105.

23 Wenger DR, Bobechko WP, Gilday DL, The spectrum of intervertebral disc-space infection in children, *J Bone Joint Surg* (1978) **60A**:100–108.

24 Boston HC, Bianco AJ, Rhodes KH, Disk space infections in children, *Orthop Clin North Am* (1975) **6**:953–964.

25 Garcia FF, Semba CP, Sartoris CC, Sartoris DJ, Diagnostic imaging of childhood spinal infection, *Orthop Rev* (1993) **22**: 321–327.

26 Eismont FJ, Bohlman HH, Prasanna LS, et al, Pyogenic and fungal vertebral osteomyelitis with paralysis, *J Bone Joint Surg* (1983) **65A**:19–29.

27   Wagner WF, The diabetic foot and amputations of the foot. In: Mann RA, ed, *Surgery of the foot*, 5th edn (CV Mosby: St Louis 1986) 421–55.

28   LeFrock JL, Joseph WS, A team approach to infections of the lower extremity in the diabetic patient, *J Foot Surg* (1987) **26**:1–2.

29   Goto Y, Horiuchi A, Kogra K, Diabetic neuropathy, *Excerpta Med Amsterdam* (1982) 11–18.

30   Joseph WS, LeFrock JL, The pathogenesis of diabetic foot infections—immunopathy, angiopathy, and neuropathy, *J Foot Surg* (1987) **26**:7–11.

31   Molenaar DM, Palumbo PJ, Wilson WR, et al, Leukocyte chemotaxis in diabetic patients and their non-diabetic first degree relatives, *Diabetes* (1976) **25**:880–883.

32   Bybee JD, Rogers DE, The phagocytic activity of polymorphonuclear leukocytes obtained from patients with diabetes mellitus, *J Lab Clin Med* (1964) **64**:1–13.

33   MacCuish AC, Urbaniak SJ, Campbell CJ, et al, Phytohaemagglutinin transformation and circulating lymphocytes of diabetic subpopulation in insulin-dependent diabetic patients, *Diabetes* (1974) **23**:708–712.

34   Kelly PJ, Bacterial arthritis in the adult, *Orthop Clin North Am* (1975) **6**:973–980.

35   Leslie BM, Harris JM, Driscoll D, Septic arthritis of the shoulder in adults, *J Bone Joint Surg* (1989) **71A**:1516–1522.

36   Sherman OH, Fox JM, Snyder SJ, et al, Arthroscopy – "No-problem surgery". An analysis of complications in two thousand six hundred and forty cases, *J Bone Joint Surg* (1986) **68–A**: 256–265

37   Burgdorfer W, Barbour AG, Hayes SF, et al, Lyme disease – a tick-borne spirochetosis? *Science* (1984) **216**:1317–1319.

38   McLaughlin TP, Zemel L, Fisher RL, et al, Chronic arthritis of the knee in Lyme disease. Review of the literature and report of two cases treated by synovectomy, *J Bone Joint Surg* (1986) **68A**:1057–1061

39   Strazzeri JC, Anzel S, Infected total hip arthroplasty due to *Actinomyces israelii* after dental extraction, a case report, *Clin Orthop* (1986) **210**:128–131.

40   Sullivan PM, Johnston RC, Kelley SS, Late infection after total hip replacement, caused by an oral organism after dental manipulation, *J Bone Joint Surg* (1990) **72A**:121–123.

41   Poss R, Thornhill TS, Ewald FC, et al, Factors influencing the incidence and outcome of infection following total joint arthroplasty, *Clin Orthop* (1984) **182**:117–126.

42   Murray RP, Bourne MH, Fitzgerald RH, Metachronous infections in patients who have had more than one total joint arthroplasty, *J Bone Joint Surg* (1991) **73A**:1469–1474

43   Inman RD, Gallegos KV, Brause BD, et al, Clinical and microbial features of prosthetic joint infection, *Am J Med* (1984) **77**:47–53.

4
DIAGNOSIS AND EVALUATION

The diagnosis of bone and joint infections is based on the clinical signs of inflammation and an accurate history. With few exceptions, the laboratory and radiographic evaluations of bone and joint infections confirm the diagnosis and identify the pathogenic organisms, thus directing antimicrobial therapy, and these evaluations are also used to monitor the progression of disease and effectiveness of therapy. Situations in which the laboratory and radiographic evaluations are important in reaching a diagnosis of infection are: when there is an associated nonunion of a long bone and when there is a loose total joint prosthesis. In addition to the proven methods of laboratory and radiographic evaluation, recent advances in biochemistry, nuclear medicine, radiology, and microbiology have added and refined the role of other methods of evaluation of bone and joint infections. This chapter reviews the salient points of: the history and physical examination; the radiographic evaluation, including diagnostic imaging; hematologic studies; and microbiological studies of material obtained by aspiration and biopsy.

History and physical examination

The history starts with the chief complaint. What led the patient to seek help? In the case of bone and joint infections this is often pain. Pain may be associated with drainage or swelling. Typically pain secondary to infection is deep seated and described as "boring or throbbing". It is not relieved by rest or inactivity, in clear distinction to pain associated with a loose total joint prosthesis or with an unhealed fracture or nonunion. Analgesics, nonsteroidal antiinflammatory drugs, and oral antibiotics may have given temporary relief from symptoms. The duration of symptoms gives some idea regarding the rate of progression. Did anything happen that may explain the onset of symptoms (eg, surgery, genitourinary instrumentation, or dental manipulation)? Frequently, there has been a prodrome of "flu like" symptoms, which is probably an effect more than the cause of the infection.

Next, a history of previous bone and joint infections is obtained. As a rule, patients with chronic bone and joint infections know when they are experiencing a flare-up. A change in the amount or character, in particular a change in the odor, of drainage may indicate malignant degeneration within the sinus tract. The existence of predisposing factors is determined (see Table 3.1, page 29). The predisposing factors encountered most frequently are peripheral vascular disease, diabetes and hemaglobinopathy. Less common predisposing factors are: inherited disorders of the immune system; intravenous drug abuse; and renal failure. Peterson and Tsukayama related various disorders of the immune system to specific infections (eg, neutrophil dysfunction and hematogenous *Staphylococcus aureus* infections of the hand).[1] Miskew et al noted the association between intravenous drug abuse and hematogenous *Pseudomonas* bone and joint infections, and specifically, spine and sacroiliac joint sepsis.[2,3] They reported 35 cases of *Pseudomonas* bone and joint infections in intravenous drug abusers. The site of infection was the spine in 13 cases, sacroiliac joint in seven, symphysis pubis in three, ischium in three, sternoclavicular joint in three, and other sites in six. Spencer noted the association between renal failure and bone and joint infections: nine patients undergoing dialysis developed hematogenous osteomyelitis, three infections of the spine, and two infections of the sternoclavicular joints.[4]

Once a history has been obtained a physical examination is performed. Symptoms secondary to a bone and joint infection are often well localized. The area is inspected for scars, sinuses and signs of inflammation: redness; swelling; and drainage. Lymph nodes are examined in the elbow, axilla, behind the knee, or in the groin. The posture of the extremity or spine is noted. Septic joints are held immobile in the position that minimizes tension on the joint capsule (eg, the knee and hip at $30°$, the hip flexed and externally rotated). Gentle palpation further localizes the symptomatic area and reveals the presence of increased temperature, and fluctuance.

Deep seated infections such as vertebral osteomyelitis, septic hip, septic shoulder, and iliac osteomyelitis are less obvious clinically and, therefore, present unique problems in diagnosis. In the case of vertebral osteomyelitis pain is elicited by gently percussing the vertebral spines. Palpation or percussion of a septic hip may not elicit pain; however, gently internally and externally rotating the hip does. Septic shoulder frequently occurs in elderly debilitated patients. Leslie et al reported a series of 18 patients with septic shoulder.[5] The diagnosis of sepsis was delayed in 14 patients. The initial diagnosis was bursitis, tendonitis, frozen shoulder, or intra-articular bleed secondary to anticoagulation. Leslie et al stress that the diagnosis of septic shoulder may not be obvious and that aspiration should be performed in questionable cases. Hematogenous iliac osteomyelitis is easily overlooked. The infection usually starts in that part of the ilium next to the sacroiliac joint and often precedes septic arthritis of that joint. Beaupre and Carroll reported 20 cases of iliac osteomyelitis.[6] Initial symptoms fell into one of three categories: buttock pain (gluteal syndrome); back hip or thigh pain (lumbar disk syndrome); or abdominal pain with signs and symptoms similar to appendicitis (abdominal syndrome). The authors found that pain elicited with compression of the pelvis and palpation of the sacroiliac joint was a reliable sign of iliac osteomyelitis. That pain localizing to the sacroiliac joint is a reliable sign of iliac osteomyelitis is supported by a report by Reilly et al.[7] In this report the final diagnosis of 17 children presenting with a painful sacroiliac joint was infection in 13. The final diagnosis in the other four patients was ankylosing spondylitis, juvenile rheumatoid arthritis, and eosinophilic granuloma of the ilium.

Radiographic evaluation

Radiographic studies used to evaluate bone and joint infections are: plain films; diagnostic imaging; computed tomography; magnetic resonance imaging; fluoroscopy and ultrasonography.

Plain films

In all cases of suspected bone and joint infection, plain films are obtained. Characteristic radiographic findings are associated with hematogenous osteomyelitis, infected fractures, spine infections, and infected arthroplasties. The radiographic signs of a septic joint are nonspecific and are limited to soft tissue swelling and intraarticular effusion.

Initial radiographic findings of acute hematogenous osteomyelitis are limited to swelling of the soft tissue over the involved metaphysis. The first radiographic finding indicating osseous involvement is one or more lytic areas surrounded by a wide area of relative radiolucency. This radiolucency indicates hyperemia of the surrounding bone. Around 10 to 14 days after the onset of infection, periosteal elevation becomes evident as osteoid laid down by the periosteum begins to calcify. Progressive layers of periosteal bone are laid down, creating an "onion skin" pattern. As the disease progresses untreated, the cortex becomes progressively more "moth eaten", with sequestered cortex appearing relatively radiodense. Eventually the entire diaphysis becomes a sequestrum surrounded by an involucrum of periosteal new bone. Radiographic findings of subacute hematogenous osteomyelitis (ie, Brodie's abscess) are a radiolucent area in the metaphysis surrounded by sclerotic or hypertrophic bone. Periosteal elevation is not present.

The clinical features of acutely infected fractures (ie, abscess formation, cellulitis, and drainage) overshadow the radiographic findings of radiolucency. Radiographic features of chronically infected fractures include: lytic areas; disorganized fluffy external callus; delayed union and nonunion; and loss of fixation.

Radiographic findings of pyogenic vertebral osteomyelitis parallel the pathophysiology, with a lag time of two to eight weeks.[8] The most frequently involved levels are from T-11 to L-5, with L-2 and L-3 leading the way. In adults, the initial finding of osteopenia localized to the superior and inferior vertebral body occurs about two weeks after the onset of infection. This is followed by a decrease in the height of the disc space around four weeks. Narrowing of the disc space is due to disc material extruding into the vertebral body, and to actual destruction of the nucleus pulposus. By 12 weeks there often is new bone formation surrounding the vertebral body, especially anteriorly. This gradually progresses to bony fusion of the vertebra anteriorly by 12 to 24 months. Radiographic findings indicating Gram negative or positive pathogens as opposed to mycotic or acid fast pathogens are: involvement of only the vertebral bodies (mycotic infections frequently involve the posterior elements);[9] absence of significant osteoporosis; destruction of the disk space, and absence of a large paraspinal mass.

Radiographic findings of an infected arthroplasty are: a progressively enlarging radiolucent zone at the bone–prosthesis interface; endosteal scalloping; and focal lytic areas. The most reliable of these is a progressively enlarging radiolucent zone. Arthroplasties which are not infected may develop a radiolucent zone at the bone–prosthesis interface. An uninfected radiolucent zone is distinguished from one due to infection in that it is less than 2 mm in width and stabilizes (ie, does not enlarge) six months following surgery. Radiographic signs of an infected arthroplasty may precede symptoms by several months. Occasionally the radiographic signs progress, and the prosthesis loosens, subsides, or even dislocates. In these cases the diagnosis is not only obvious radiographically but also invariably clinically.[10,11]

Diagnostic imaging

Diagnostic imaging techniques are used to evaluate bone and joint infections. In all types of diagnostic imaging, the patient is injected with a radioactive pharmaceutical. Following a suitable period of time, areas of radioactive pharmaceutical concentration are found by scanning the patient with a gamma camera. The two major disadvantages of diagnostic imaging are: that the images lack resolution; and that the radiopharmaceuticals are also concentrated in noninfected areas, ie, they are nonspecific. Despite these disadvantages diagnostic imaging often provides information concerning the extent of infection, and previously unidentified foci of infection. Diagnostic imaging can be valuable in the evaluation of questionably infected total joints and nonunions.

There are three radionuclides commonly used in diagnostic imaging: technetium-99, used as the methylene diphosphate (Tc-99); gallium-67 (Ga-67); and indium-111 (In-111). These three radionuclides have different characteristics which make them useful in particular settings. Tc-99, immediately after injection, is limited to the intravascular space, where it is partially protein bound. A scan in this "immediate" phase indicates the amount of blood flow to a specific area. Within 15 minutes the concentration of Tc-99 in the intravascular space has equilibrated with the concentration in the extravascular space. A scan obtained in this "early" phase may indicate hyperemia. One of the most common causes of hyperemia is cellulitis. Following the early phase, the amount of Tc-99 continues to decrease in the vascular space because of uptake by bone and excretion by the kidneys. Tc-99 binds to collagen in areas of osteoblastic activity. At four to six hours approximately 40% of the Tc-99 has been excreted by the kidneys; the remaining 60% is bound to the bone. A scan obtained in this "delayed" phase may reflect increased osteoblastic activity, not hypervascularity. Any process that disturbs the normal balance of bone production and resorption can produce an abnormal delayed bone scan. In an uncompromised bone, a negative bone scan with Tc-99 rules out hematogenous osteomyelitis, as the bone scan becomes abnormal within hours to days following the onset of infection. An increased accumulation of the radionuclide or a "hot" lesion reflects the degree of reactive new

bone formation as well as increased blood flow. "Cold" or photon deficient areas are less common but may represent osteomyelitis, particularly in the early stages. Decreased uptake in these areas is caused by a variety of factors including: inadequate blood supply due to a subperiosteal abscess or vasospasm; a rapidly progressive lytic lesion of the bone; or an infarct.

Sequential or dynamic bone imaging denotes scanning the patient in the immediate, early, and delayed phases. Because sequential scans compare changes in count accumulation, they are a more specific measure of an inflammatory processes than static scans obtained only in the delayed phase. When sequentially scanned, osteomyelitis is characterized by an increased count accumulation in all phases; soft tissue infections have an increased count accumulation in the early phase, but the delayed phase is relatively cold. Other noninfectious processes (eg, posttraumatic arthritis) have decreased count accumulation in the early phase and increased in the delayed phase.

Ga-67 is used primarily to localize areas of inflammation.[12] The mechanism of uptake in these areas is not entirely clear. To a greater or lesser extent Ga-67 binds to: leukocytes, which migrate to sites of inflammation; transferrin and lactoferrin, proteins which are found at the site of inflammation; and the microorganisms themselves. Ga-67 scans are usually obtained in conjunction with Tc-99 scans. The Tc-99 scan is performed at four hours, the Ga-67 scan at 48 hours. A Ga-67 scan which is congruent and hotter than the Tc-99 scan is indicative of infection. A noncongruent scan or a Ga-67 scan which is colder than the Tc-99 scan indicates that infection is not present.

In-111 is used to label leukocytes. In order to do this, the leukocytes are separated from approximately 100 ml of blood obtained from the patient. The cells are labeled with In-111 and injected into the patient. These cells then travel to areas of inflammation, which are localized by scanning. Because In-111 uptake is limited to areas to which leukocytes have migrated it holds more promise than either Tc-99 or Ga-67 in the diagnosis of infection, particularly when the infection is posttraumatic or postsurgical.

Diagnostic imaging is most useful in five clinical settings: the diagnosis of subclinical or latent osteomyelitis; the diagnosis of osteomyelitis in children; the diagnosis of occult infection; the differentiation of infection from bone infarct; and the diagnosis of infected total joint prosthesis.

Esterhai et al investigated the accuracy of In-111 scanning in the detection of subclinical osteomyelitis in association with nonunion.[13] In their study the patient was first scanned and then the suspect area was biopsied. The authors found that the scans were 100% accurate, sensitive, and specific. Other studies have confirmed high accuracy, sensitivity and specificity of In-111 scans in the diagnosis of subclinical musculoskeletal infections. Nepola et al reported a large series of nonunions with possible infection.[14] They found a low incidence of false negatives (ie, if the scan was negative the chance that there was osteomyelitis was very low). Merkel et al studied 50 patients with suspected subclinical musculoskeletal sepsis.[15,16] They found that the In-111 labeled leukocyte technique was 83% accurate and sensitive; in comparison the sequential Tc-99 and Ga-67 technique had an accuracy of only 57%. Magnuson et al confirmed these results in a similar study from the same institution.[17]

Tc-99 scans are of value in diagnosing pediatric osteomyelitis. Howie et al reported a series in which a Tc-99 scan correctly indicated the diagnosis of osteomyelitis in 55 of 62 infected sites, and was correctly negative in 74 of 79 children.[18] The authors point out that Tc-99 scans are very inaccurate in the diagnosis of septic joints.

Attempts have been made to localize occult infections of the spine and pelvis with diagnostic imaging. In-111 labeled leukocyte scans have not proven to be useful in the detection of occult spine infection.[19] Beaupre and Carroll found Tc-99 scans extremely useful in the diagnosis of iliac osteomyelitis.[6]

Differentiating a bone infarct from hematogenous osteomyelitis is difficult. This problem arises most frequently in patients with hemaglobinopathies, but also in patients with Gaucher's disease.[20,21] The problem is made worse in that the symptoms of bone infarct and osteomyelitis are similar (ie, pain and swelling), the laboratory evaluation may be identical (ie, elevated ESR and white count), and an open biopsy is performed only if necessary, because of the risk of introducing bacteria into an infarcted bone. Diagnostic imaging can be invaluable in this setting. Amundson et al were able to distinguish between bone infarct and infection in patients with sickle cell anemia by using Tc-99 and Ga-67 scans.[22] In contrast, Mallouh and Talab found that although bone scans were useful in some cases they were not always diagnostic.[23] Bell et al found that a cold delayed Tc-99 scan is virtually diagnostic of bone infarct and rules out infection in patients with Gaucher's disease.[20]

The differentiation of a loose total joint prosthesis from an infected prosthesis is crucial, and it is on this area that many reports focus. Rand and Brown and Palestro et al reported series of patients with loose or infected knee and hip arthroplasties.[24,25] In both studies the In-111 labeled leukocyte scans identified infection with an accuracy and sensitivity of about 80%. In contrast, Wukich et al found that while In-111 labeled leukocyte scans were sensitive (ie, there were no false negatives in their series of 24 patients with possible infected arthroplasties) they were not accurate (there were ten false positives).[26]

Single photon emission computed tomography (SPECT) adds another wrinkle to diagnostic imaging. In this technique, following administration of a radiopharmaceutical, a set of images is generated by a gamma camera which moves in an orbit around the region of interest. Tomographic reconstruction by a computer results in images that reflect the three dimensional distribution of the radiopharmaceutical. This technique potentially offers more information than planar images obtained with routine bone scans. Its importance has not yet been verified in clinical trials.

Summary

Diagnostic imaging is usually a reliable method of diagnosing infection; In-111 labeled leukocyte scans alone are probably more accurate than Tc-99 and Ga-67 scans, but there is tremendous variation in the accuracy of In-111 scans from institution to institution. In the final analysis, any condition that affects bone metabolism or vascularity (eg, arthritis; successfully treated or chronic osteomyelitis; fracture; previous surgery; infarct; neoplasm; prosthetic loosening; and peripheral vascular disease) potentially alter radionuclide uptake. Therefore, bone scans must be interpreted along with clinical signs and other diagnostic procedures.

Computed tomography

Computed tomography (CT) scanning involves passing numerous narrow X-ray beams through the area to be scanned. The amount of X-ray transmission is determined by the attenuating properties of the tissues through which these beams pass. The amount of X-ray transmission recorded and analyzed in such a way that cross-sectional images are produced. These cross-sectional images can be combined to produce three dimensional images. Three dimensional CT imaging methods are used in the evaluation of traumatic disorders of anatomically complex regions of the body such as the spine, pelvis, hip, shoulder, and facial bones.

CT is the most effective method of defining intracortical abnormalities and of detecting calcification or ossification. The early CT findings of infection include increased marrow density. This may be subtle because of the attenuation from surrounding cortical bone. In chronic osteomyelitis CT scanning may indicate sclerosis, demineralization, periosteal reaction, and sequestra. CT scans are useful in the evaluation of spine infections to determine whether there are soft tissue abscesses.

Magnetic resonance imaging

Magnetic resonance imaging (MRI) is capable of generating high quality sectional representations of the human body at any angle or perspective. It provides both anatomic and physiologic data, without the use of ionizing radiation. The distribution of hydrogen is currently used as the basis of MRI and the differences in tissue contrast are based on differences in proton density, T_1 relaxation rates, T_2 relaxation rates, blood flow among tissues, and the particular pulse sequence selected.

MRI is important in the diagnosis of spine disorders. It indicates the exact anatomic location of vertebral and paravertebral tuberculous abscesses and is, therefore, helpful in the preoperative evaluation and in monitoring the response to therapy.

Klein et al compared MRI, CT and Tc-99 bone scans in the diagnosis of septic sacroiliac joints.[27] They found that MRI gave the diagnosis more quickly and more accurately localized the precise site of infection.

MRI has been used to distinguish cellulitis from abscesses and to indicate if either has progressed to involve neighboring bone (Figs 4.1 and 4.2). This is important in arriving at a rational treatment plan (antibiotics alone for cellulitis versus débridement and antibiotics for an abscess and osteomyelitis). Wang et al used MRI to study a series of diabetic patients with foot infections.[28] They found that the sensitivity of MRI was 98% and plain films 52%. Mason et al found that MRI accurately diagnosed and predicted the extent of disease in 14 patients with possible osteomyelitis of the lower extremity.[29] The authors conclude that their study "has shown that MRI appears to be a promising

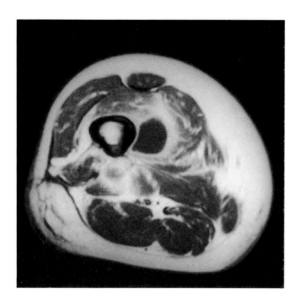

Figure 4.1

T1 weighted image of the thigh indicating a large fluid collection medial to the femur, loss of tissue planes, and increased water content (inflammation) of surrounding soft tissue.

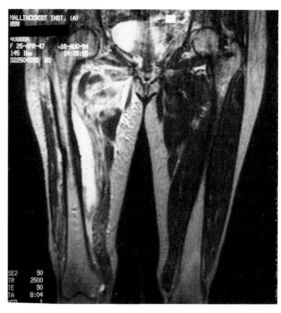

Figure 4.2

T2 weighted image of the same patient indicating a large fluid collection medial to the femur.

modality in the detection of osteomyelitis superimposed on chronic tissue changes of old infection, trauma, and surgery".

Gadolinium-diethylenetriamine pentaacetic acid (Gd-DPTA) is a paramagnetic contrast medium which increases lesion contrast in neoplastic disease of brain and spine. It is potentially a valuable adjunct to noncontrast MRI in the diagnosis of spine infection, but it requires further study.

Ultrasonography

Ultrasonographic images are produced by the reflection or refraction of sound waves as they encounter interfaces between tissues of different acoustic impedances. Lesions are characterized as being either cystic or solid. The advantage of ultrasound is that it is noninvasive, painless and does not expose the patient to ionizing radiation. It is generally less expensive and more rapidly performed than alternative studies.

Ultrasound can distinguish cellulitis from abscesses, normal periosteum from periosteum elevated by an abscess and a normal joint from one with an effusion. Because it allows localization of lesions in three dimensions, ultrasonography is a useful technique for guiding percutaneous aspiration or biopsy.

Hematologic studies

The two hematologic studies obtained most frequently are a differential cell count and the erythrocyte sedimentation rate (ESR). In most chronic bone and joint infections the differential cell count is within the limits of normal. When the differential cell count is abnormal it indicates the host response to infection. An elevated white cell count with an increase in the proportion of polymorphonuclear leukocytes is one of the hallmarks of a bacterial infection. An increase in numbers of monocytes is found with tuberculous and fungal infections. An increase in lymphocytes may indicate a viral infection, or a chronic infection.

The ESR is defined as the distance that a column of erythrocytes sediments in one hour.[30] This distance is increased by aggregation of the erythrocytes because as the aggregate, or rouleau, increases in size its weight relative to its surface area increases. Increased tendency to form rouleaus is based not upon changes in the red blood cells, but rather changes in the plasma proteins. The red blood cells have negative charges and therefore normally repel each other. In the presence of infection there is an increased concentration of positively charged plasma proteins (eg, acute phase proteins and fibrinogen), resulting in increased rouleau formation and an increased ESR.

There are two methods used to determine the ESR: the Westergren method and the Wintrobe and Landsberg method.[31,32] The upper limit of normal for the Westergren method is 16 mm for men and 25 mm for women. The respective upper limits of normal for the Wintrobe and Landsberg method is 6 mm and 16 mm. Conditions that lower the ESR include administration of steroids and nonsteroidal antiinflammatory drugs, hemaglobinopathies such as sickle cell disease, leukemia and polycythemia. Conditions that elevate the ESR are inflammation due to infection or collagen vascular disease, surgery, pregnancy, and tumors.

In the clinical situations of an infected arthroplasty and vertebral osteomyelitis the ESR is valuable in the diagnosis and monitoring of the therapeutic response. Thoren and Wigren studied patients with infected or loose hip arthroplasties.[33] They found that an ESR greater than 35 mm/h in patients without an underlying disease is indicative of infection. In patients with an underlying disease a 50% increase of the preoperative ESR six months following an arthroplasty indicated the presence of infection. Wisneski used a similar approach in a group of patients with vertebral osteomyelitis.[34] He found that in patients with an elevated ESR, a 33% decrease from the pretherapy ESR indicated a good response to medical therapy.

Microbiological studies

The pathologic organisms are isolated by incubating, in appropriate culture media, material obtained from the infected area by: surface swabs; aspiration; or biopsy. When the pathologic organisms have been isolated, their sensitivity to various antibiotics is determined in vitro. The pattern of sensitivity directs antibiotic therapy.

Isolation of organisms

The importance of isolating all pathogenic organisms in a bone and joint infection cannot be overemphasized. In contrast to clean cases (in which five or more colony forming units must be isolated before the diagnosis of infection is made) all organisms isolated from an infected area by one of these techniques are assumed to be pathogens.[35] The importance of distinguishing patients with clinical signs of infection from those without signs of infection is underlined by a study reported by Dobbins et al.[36] They cultured implants retrieved from asymptomatic patients, and found bacteria in 28% of cases. This demonstrates that adherent bacteria can exist for years in a dormant state on implants without evoking the clinical signs of infection.

Wound swabs, aspiration, and biopsy are the possible techniques of obtaining material from which pathogenic organisms can be cultured. Prior to obtaining material for culture it is essential to discontinue all antibiotics for at least one month. This insures that specific species of bacteria will not be suppressed and therefore not identified.[37] The relative accuracy of wound swabs, aspiration, and percutaneous biopsy is important. Swabs of wounds or sinus tracts fell into disrepute following a report by Mackowiack et al in 1978.[38] Their study included a large number of patients with chronic diabetic ulcers of the foot. While wound swabs may not be accurate in this group of patients, I believe that they are accurate in other settings, such as posttraumatic or postsurgical osteomyelitis. We reported a series of patients with posttraumatic osteomyelitis who underwent a percutaneous biopsy, surgical débridement, and, if they were draining, a swab of the wound.[39] We compared the accuracy of these three methods of obtaining material for culture. We found that: the most accurate method of identifying all the pathogenic organisms was to obtain numerous cultures throughout the surgical débridement; cultures of material obtained by swabbing of the superficial aspect of the wound or the sinus identified 90% of the pathogens isolated during surgical débridement; and percutaneous biopsy of patients with latent osteomyelitis (ie, a patient with a clear history of osteomyelitis but no signs of infection at the time of examination) was of no value in ruling out latent infection. I assume that the lack of sensitivity of percutaneous biopsies is due to the fact that the infected area is not homogenous. Different organisms may be growing in isolated microenvironments, and, therefore, there is a high probability that a needle biopsy will miss some of these microenvironments.[40,41]

Aspiration denotes retrieval of fluid through a needle, and is distinct from a biopsy, in which tissue is obtained. Aspiration is used to diagnose the presence of an abscess, to obtain material for culture, and to manage infected joints.[42] White blood cell counts of greater than 70,000/ml indicate a septic joint. Gram stain of the synovial fluid may indicate pathogenic organisms and fluid is sent for culture. Diagnostic criteria for immunocompromised patients (ie, those with malignant neoplasms; taking steroids; with acquired immune deficiency; or intravenous drug abusers) are different.[43] In these patients, a synovial fluid white blood cell count of 20,000 cells/ml or greater indicates infectious arthritis unless there are other causes of inflammatory arthropathy. Ancillary studies such as serum and synovial glucose concentrations, ESR and differential synovial fluid cell count (increased monocytes and lymphocytes point toward fungal or mycobacterial infections) help in arriving at a diagnosis prior to cultures being positive. If all routine cultures are negative and suspicion of infection is still high, special care and culture techniques for *Haemophilus influenzae*, gonococci, anaerobes, fungi and mycobacteria are undertaken. Esterhai and Gelb found that only 10% of routine cultures of fluid aspirated from joints infected with gonococcus were positive.[44] In this same study, blood cultures were positive in 50% of patients with nongonococcal septic arthritis and 10% of patients with gonococcal septic arthritis.

Routine aspiration of an arthroplasty prior to revision is controversial. Barrack and Harris reported a series of 270 patients who underwent radiographically directed aspiration prior to revision hip arthroplasty.[45] They found an incidence of false positive results of 13% and a remarkably low incidence of true positive results of 6%. In a similar study, Gould et al reported a series of 78 patients with a potentially infected hip prosthesis.[46] All 78 underwent radiographically directed aspiration followed by revision arthroplasty. Like Barrack and Harris's report, there was low sensitivity and accuracy of the aspiration in the diagnosis of infection. Cucler et al went even further in their report of 43 patients with a possible infected total joint arthroplasty.[47] They concluded that a perioperative evaluation consisting of ESR, In-111 labeled leukocyte scan, and aspiration for culture and sensitivity will fail to

_ .ect the presence of sepsis in approximately 25% of cases of actual infection. The authors of these studies conclude that aspiration should be performed only if there is tangible clinical evidence of infection, and not on a routine basis. In complete contradistinction, Roberts et al reported the results of essentially the same study (ie, aspiration followed by revision hip arthroplasty).[48] They found the incidence of true positive results to be 94% and the incidence of false positive results to be 5%. The conflicting results of these studies is explained by the obvious care with which Roberts et al performed their aspirations (eg, use of blood culture bottles for transport of material and immediate plating of the material). Based upon these studies, in cases in which revision arthroplasty is being contemplated, aspiration of the joint should be limited to those patients with clinical and laboratory findings indicative of infection (ie, pain, history of infection, fever, elevated ESR, and increased white blood cell count). In cases in which aspiration is performed, the technical details are important in achieving an accurate result. However, failure to culture organisms from material obtained by biopsy or aspiration does not exclude infection, and even if cultures are positive, all the pathogens may not have been isolated.

Biopsy implies harvesting of tissue. Biopsies are taken prior to surgery by the technique of percutaneous biopsy or during surgical débridement. In the technique of percutaneous biopsy, a large hollow needle is used to obtain tissue for culture and histologic examination. In my experience Craig or Ackerman needles facilitate the procedure. In the spine, the nucleotome (an instrument used for percutaneous spinal disc excision) provides good samples for histologic examination and culture and at the same time the majority of infected material can be removed. In anatomically remote areas, such as the spine, sacroiliac joint, and hip, or in cases in which a small nidus is to be biopsied, fluoroscopy, CT scanning or ultrasonography are utilized to insure accuracy.[49,50]

When débriding a bone and joint infection, material for culture is obtained throughout the procedure from several different areas. Material is sent for aerobic, anaerobic, fungal and mycobacterial culture. In addition to cultures, during revision surgery for an infected arthroplasty, tissue is obtained for intraoperative Gram stain and frozen section. The presence of white blood cells or bacteria indicate persistent infection. When débriding a chronically infected wound, tissue from the sinus tract is obtained for histologic examination to rule out malignant degeneration.

Antibiotic sensitivities

The method used most frequently to determine the sensitivity of a strain of bacteria to a given antibiotic is the disc diffusion technique.[51] In this method commercially available filter paper discs impregnated with specific quantities of drug are laid on the surface of agar plates over which a culture of the microorganism has been streaked. At 18 hours the plate is reexamined. If the organism is sensitive to the antibiotic on the filter paper disc there is a clear zone around the disc. The size of this clear zone is interpreted as indicating that the bacteria are susceptible, intermediately susceptible, or resistant to the antibiotic being tested.[52] This method has the advantage that it is simple and inexpensive. However, it provides only qualitative data. Quantitative data are provided by methods based on serial dilutions of antibiotics in broth which contains a culture of the test microorganism. The lowest concentration of antibiotic that prevents growth after 18 to 24 hours is known as the minimal inhibitory concentration (MIC). The lowest concentration that sterilizes the medium is known as the minimal bactericidal concentration (MBC).[53] Schlicter and MacLean described serum peak and trough bacteriostatic and bactericidal levels.[54] These levels are determined by incubating pathogenic bacteria in serial dilutions of the patient's serum which have been obtained immediately prior to and immediately following antibiotic administration. Serum bacteriostatic and bactericidal levels have the disadvantage that they are difficult to obtain and that they vary widely from laboratory to laboratory. In general MICs and MBCs are adequate for the management of bone and joint infections.

Despite the fact that we determine antibiotic therapy based upon in vitro MICs, they are not necessarily relevant or accurate. The concept of bacteria existing in two phases, having different susceptibilities to antibiotics and to host defense mechanisms, explains much of what we see in vitro and clinically. MICs are determined from floating bacteria and thus may give an unrealistically optimistic picture of susceptibility.[55] Widmer et al found that there was no correlation with the MICs of the pathogenic organism to the antibiotic being administered and the clinical outcome.[56] They speculated that this is due to the different susceptibilities of floating and adherent bacteria. Bacteria on implanted biomaterials are commonly resistant to antibiotic levels well above permissible therapeutic levels.[40,41,57] Glycocalyx plays an important role in this resistance by directly suppressing phagocytosis of bacteria by PMNs,[58] and because adherent bacteria are metabolically inert.[59] This would mean that sterilization of infected implants may depend on antibiotics which kill stationary phase and adherent bacteria. Despite the importance of glycocalyx, there is no reliable assay for its production.

References

1   Peterson PK, Tsukayama DT, Bone and joint infections in immunocompromised patients. In: Gustillo RB, Gruninger RP, Tsukayama DT, eds, *Orthopaedic infection: diagnosis and treatment* (WB Saunders: Philadelphia 1989) 81–60.

2   Miskew DBW, Lorenz MA, Pearson RL, et al, Pseudomonas aeruginosa bone and joint infection in drug abusers, *J Bone Joint Surg* (1983) **65A**:829–832.

3   Miskew DBW, Block RA, Witt PF, Aspiration of the sacroiliac joints, *J Bone Joint Surg* (1971) **61A**:1071–1072.

4   Spencer JD, Bone and joint infection in a renal unit, *J Bone Joint Surg* (1986) **68B**:489–493.

5   Leslie BM, Harris JM, Driscoll D, Septic arthritis of the shoulder in adults, *J Bone Joint Surg* (1989) **71A**:1516–1521.

6   Beaupre A, Carroll N, The syndromes of iliac osteomyelitis in children, *J Bone Joint Surg* (1979) **61A**:1087–1092.

7   Reilly JP, Gross RH, Emans JB, et al, Disorders of the sacro-iliac joint in children, *J Bone Joint Surg* (1988) **70A**:31–40.

8   Digby JM, Kersley JB, Pyogenic non-tubercular spinal infection, *J Bone Joint Surg* (1979) **61B**:47.

9   Griffith HED, Jones DM, Pyogenic infection of the spine, *J Bone Joint Surg* (1971) **53B**:383–391.

10   Bergstrom B, Lindgren L, Lindberg L, Radiographic abnormalities caused by postoperative infection following total hip arthroplasty, *Clin Orthop Rel Res* (1974) **99**:95–102.

11   Carlson A, Eglund N, Gentz C, et al, Radiographic loosening after revision with gentamicin-containing cement for deep infection in total hip arthroplasties, *Clin Orthop Rel Res* (1985) **194**:271–279.

12   Propst-Proctor SL, Dillingham MF, McDougall RI, et al, The white blood scan in orthopedics, *Clin Orthop Rel Res* (1982) **168**:157–165.

13   Esterhai JL, Goll SR, McCarthy KE, et al, Indium-111 leukocyte scintigraphic detection of

subclinical osteomyelitis complicating delayed and nonunion long bone fractures: a prospective study, *J Orthop Res* (1987) 5:1–6.

14 Nepola JV, Seabold JE, Marsh JL, et al, Diagnosis of infection in ununited fractures, *J Bone Joint Surg* (1993) **75A**:1816–1822.

15 Merkel KD, Brown ML, Dewanjee MK, et al, Comparison of indium-labeled leukocyte imaging with sequential technetium-gallium scanning in the diagnosis of low grade musculoskeletal sepsis, *J Bone Joint Surg* (1985) **67A**:465–476.

16 Merkel KD, Fitzgerald RH, Brown ML, Scitigraphic evaluation in musculo sepsis, *Orthop Clin North Am* (1984) **15**:401–416.

17 Magnuson JE, Brown ML, Hauser MF, et al, In-111-labeled leukocyte scintigraphy in suspected orthopedic prosthesis infection: comparison with other imaging modalities, *Radiology* (1988) **168**:235–239.

18 Howie DW, Savage JP, Wilson TG, et al, The technetium phosphate bone scan in the diagnosis of osteomyelitis in childhood, *J Bone Joint Surg* (1983) **65A**:431–437.

19 Whalen JL, Brown ML, McLeod R, et al, Limitations of indium leukocyte imaging for the diagnosis of spine infections, *Spine* (1991) **16**:193–197.

20 Bell RS, Mankin HJ, Doppelt SH, Osteomyelitis in gaucher disease, *J Bone Joint Surg* (1986) **68A**:1380–1387.

21 Epps CH, Bryant DD, Coles MJ, Osteomyelitis in patients who have sickle-cell disease. Diagnosis and management, *J Bone Joint Surg* (1991) **73A**:1281–1294.

22 Amundson TR, Siegel MJ, Siegel BA, Osteomyelitis and infarction in sickle-cell hemaglobinopathies: differentiation by combined technetium and gallium scintigraphy, *Radiology* (1984) **53**:807–812.

23 Mallouh A, Talab Y, Bone and joint infections in patients with sickle cell disease, *J Pediat Orthop* (1985) **5**:158–162.

24 Rand JA, Brown ML, The value of indium 111 leukocyte scanning in the evaluation of painful or infected total knee arthroplasties, *Clin Orthop Rel Res* (1990) **259**:179–182.

25 Palestro CJ, Swyer AJ, Kim CK, Infected knee prosthesis: diagnosis with In-111 leukocyte, Tc99–m sulfur colloid, and Tc-99m-MDP imaging, *Radiology* (1991) **179**:645–648.

26 Wukich DK, Abreu SH, Callaghan JJ, et al, Diagnosis of infection by preoperative scintigraphy with indium labeled white blood cells, *J Bone Joint Surg* (1987) **69A**:1353–1360.

27 Klein MA, Winalski CS, Wax MR, et al, MR imaging of septic sacroiliitis, *J Comp Assist Tomogr* (1991) **15**:126–132.

28 Wang A, Weinstein D, Greenfield L, et al, MRI and diabetic foot infections, *MRI* (1990) **8**:805–809.

29 Mason MD, Zlatkin MB, Esterhai JL, et al, Chronic complicated osteomyelitis of the lower extremity: evaluation with MR imaging, *Radiology* (1989) **173**:355–359.

30 Covey DC, Albright JA, Current concepts review: clinical significance of the erythrocyte sedimentation rate in orthopedic surgery, *J Bone Joint Surg* (1987) **69A**:148–151.

31 Westergren A, The technique of the red cell sedimentation reaction, *Am Rev Tuberc* (1926) **14**:94–101.

32 Wintrobe MM, Landsberg JW, A standardized technique for the blood sedimentation test, *Am J Med Sci* (1935) **189**:102–115.

33 Thoren B, Wigren A, Erythrocyte sedimentation rate in infection of total hip replacements, *Orthopedics* (1991) **14**:495–497.

34 Wisneski RJ, Infectious disease of the spine, diagnostic and treatment considerations, *Orthop Clin North Am* (1991) **22**:491–501.

35 Dietz FR, Koontz FP, Found EM, et al, The importance of positive bacterial cultures of specimens obtained during clean orthopedic operations, *J Bone Joint Surg* (1991) **73A**:1200–1207.

36 Dobbins JJ, Seligson D, Raff MJ, Bacterial colonization of orthopedic devices in the absence of clinical infection, *J Inf Dis* (1988) **158**:203.

37 Windsor RE, Management of total knee arthroplasty infection, *Orthop Clin North Am* (1991) **3**:531–538.

38 Mackowiak PA, Jones SR, Smith JW, Diagnostic value of sinus tract cultures in chronic osteomyelitis, *JAMA* (1978) **239**:2772–2775.

39 Perry CR, Pearson RL, Miller GA, Accuracy of cultures of material from swabbing of the superficial aspect of the wound and needle biopsy in the preoperative assessment of osteomyelitis, *J Bone Joint Surg* (1991) **5**:745–749.

40 Costerton JW, The etiology of cryptic bacterial infections: a hypothesis, *Rev Infect Dis* (1984) **6**:608–616.

41 Marrie TJ, Costerton JW, Mode of growth of bacterial pathogens in chronic polymicrobial human osteomyelitis, *J Clin Microb* (1985) **22**:924–933.

42 McCutchan HJ, Fisher RC, Synovial leukocytosis in infectious arthritis, *Clin Orthop Rel Res* (1990) **257**:226–230.

43 Brennan PJ, Pia DeGirolamo M, Musculoskeletal infections in immunocompromised hosts, *Orthop Clin North Am* (1991) **3**:389–399.

44 Esterhai JL, Gelb I, Adult septic arthritis, *Orthop Clin North Am* (1991) **3**:503–514.

45 Barrack RL, Harris WH, The value of aspiration of the hip joint before revision total hip arthroplasty, *J Bone Joint Surg* (1993) **75A**:66–76.

46 Gould ES, Potter HG, Bober SE, Role of routine percutaneous hip aspirations prior to prosthesis revision, *Skeletal Radiol* (1990) **19**:427–430.

47 Cucler JM, Star AM, Alavi A, et al, Diagnosis and management of the infected total joint arthroplasty, *Orthop Clin North Am* (1991) **3**:523–530.

48 Roberts P, Walters AJ, McMinn DJW, Diagnosing infection in hip replacements, *J Bone Joint Surg* (1992) **74B**:265–269.

49 Miskew DB, Block RA, Witt PF, Aspiration of infected sacro-iliac joints, *J Bone Joint Surg* (1979) **61A**:1071–1072.

50 Yu WY, Siu C, Wing PC, et al, Percutaneous suction aspiration for osteomyelitis, *Spine* (1991) **2**:198–202.

51 Bauer AW, Kirby WMM, Sherris JC, et al, Antibiotic susceptibility testing by a standardized single disc method, *Am J Clin Pathol* (1966) **45**:493–496.

52 National Committee for Clinical Laboratory Standards, *Methods for dilution antimicrobial susceptibility tests for bacteria that grow aerobically* (Villanova, Pennsylvania: NCCLS 1983).

53 Ericcson HM, Sherris JC, Antibiotic sensitivity testing. Report of an international collaborative study, *Acta Pathol Microbiol Scand* (1971) **227**:1.

54 Schlicter JG, MacLean H, A method of determining the effective therapeutic level in the treatment of subacute bacterial endocarditis with penicillin, *Am Heart J* (1947) **34**:209.

55 Naylor PT, Myrvik QN, Gristina A, Antibiotic resistance of biomaterial-adherent coagulase-positive staphylococci, *Clin Orthop Rel Res* (1990) **261**:126–133.

56 Widmer AF, Colombo VE, Gachter A, Salmonella infection in total hip replacement: tests to predict the outcome of antimicrobial therapy, *Scand J Infect Dis* (1990) **22**:611–618.

57 Oga M, Arizona T, Sugioka Y, Bacterial adherence to bioinert and bioactive materials studied in vitro, *Acta Orthop Scand* (1993) **63**:273–276.

58 Veringa EM, Ferguson DA, Lambe DW, et al, The role of glycocalyx in surface phagocytosis of bacteroides spp. in the presence and abscence of clindamycin, *J Antimicrob Chemother* (1989) **23**:711–720.

59 Nickel JC, Rusescka I, Wright JB, et al, Tobramycin resistance of pseudomonas aeruginosa cells growing as a biofilm on urinary catheter material, *Antimicrob Agents Chemother* (1985) **27**:619–624

5
NONOPERATIVE MANAGEMENT

Nonoperative management of bone and joint infections consists of the following techniques: administration of antibiotics systemically or locally; maximization of the systemic physiologic status of the patient; stimulation by electrical and magnetic fields; and application of hyperbaric oxygen.

Antibiotic therapy – systemic

The important parameters of systemic antibiotic therapy are: selection of the antibiotic; documentation of systemic levels; and duration of therapy.

Selection of systemic antibiotic

When antibiotics are first initiated in patients with bone and joint infections the pathogenic organisms frequently have not yet been identified. Antibiotic selection is based upon the clinician's guess as to the identity of the most likely organism. This guess is based upon previous cultures or various risk factors (see Chapter 2).

Occasionally the patient is extremely ill, or the infectious process is progressing rapidly. In these circumstances, antibiotics are administered which will cover all possible pathogens (Table 5.1). Eventually, appropriate antibiotic therapy depends on the isolation and identification of all pathogenic organisms. Any organism present at the site of infection is assumed to be a pathogen. This includes organisms commonly considered to be contaminants, ie, *Staphylococcus epidermidis* and *diphtheroides*. When all pathogens have been identified, antibiotic selection is based on the sensitivies of the organisms and the potential toxicity of the antibiotic. Table 5.2 lists the organisms commonly encountered as pathogens in bone and joint infections and the most commonly utilized antibiotics. Precise identification of the pathogenic organism requires that material be obtained for culture. It is key that this is done prior to administering antibiotics. Once antibiotics have been administered, even resistant organisms may fail to grow in culture. The one exception to this rule is hematogenous spine infections, or discitis, in children. This is because the pathogenic organism is invariably *Staphylococcus aureus*. Biopsy of the disc is performed only when there is no response to systemic antibiotic therapy.[1]

Table 5.1 Empirical antibacterial therapy for osteomyelitis on clinical grounds (optimal antimicrobial therapy is based upon accurate identification and in vitro susceptibility testing of causal agents; these are only "initial" guidelines)

Modifying circumstances	Etiologies	Suggested regimen
Newborn	*Staphylococcus aureus* Enterobacteriaceae Group A, B streptococci	Pencillinase resistant synthetic penicillin
Child ≤4 years	*H. influenzae* Streptococci *Staphylococcus aureus*	Parenteral 3rd generation cephalosporin
Child >4 years	*Staphylococcus aureus* Streptococci *H. influenzae*	Clindamycin or vancomycin
Adult (including history of drug abuse)	*Staphylococcus aureus* (occasional Enterobacteriaceae, *Streptococcus* sp.)	Pencillinase resistant synthetic penicillin (if Gram negative bacilli on smear, add parenteral 3rd generation cephalosporin)
Postoperative or posttrauma	*Staphylococcus aureus* Enterobacteriaceae *Pseudomonas* sp.	2nd generation cephalosporin, vancomycin + parenteral 3rd generation cephalosporin or imipenem cilastatin
Nail puncture, foot	*Pseudomonas* sp.	Ciprofloxacin, ticarcillin clavulanate, imipenem or parenteral 3rd generation cephalosporin
Contiguous with decubitus ulcer, diabetic foot	Polymicrobic: aerobic cocci, baccili + anaerobes	Clindamycin, cephalexin

Table 5.2 Antimicrobial agents of choice against selected organisms

Bacterial species	Recommended	Alternative	Also effective (comments)
Clostridium tetani, perfringene	Penicillin G	Doxycycline	Erythrocmycin, chloramphenicol, cefazolin, cefoxitin, antipseudomonal β-lactamase susceptible penicillins Bacitracin (p.o)
Clostridium difficile	Vancomycin	Ciprofloxacin	
Corynebacterium jekeium	Erythromycin	Penicillin	Clindamycin, rifampin
Corynebacterium diphtheriae	"	"	"
Edwardsiella tarda	Ampicillin	Cephalothin	Antipseudomonal aminoglycosidic antibiotics, chloramphenicol, ciprofloxacin
Enterobacteriaceae	Imipenem or antipseudomonal aminoglycoside	Ticarcillin clavulanate or ciprofloxacin	
Enterococcus faecalis	Ampicillin + gentamicin	Vancomycin + gentamicin	
Enterococcus faecium (high level gentamicin, vancomycin resistance)	Ciprofloxacin + gentamicin + rifampin		Experience limited to a few cases
Eikenella corrodens	Penicillin G or ampicillin	Erythromycin	Doxycycline, cefoxitin, cefotaxime, imipenem (clindamycin resistant)
Escherichia coli	Dependent upon site of infection – most agents except penicillinase resistant synthetic penicillin		
Haemophilus influenzae	Amoxicillin clavulanate, oral 2nd or 3rd generation cephalosporins, trimethoprim/ sulfamethoxazole	Imipenem, ciprofloxacin	
Morganella sp.	Imipenem or parenteral 3rd generation cephalosporin	Ciprofloxacin, aztreonam	Antipseudomonal aminoglycoside

Table 5.2 (contd)

Bacterial species	Recommended	Alternative	Also effective (comments)
Neisseria gonorrhoeae	Ceftriaxone	Spectinomycin, cefixime, fluoroquinolones	Ampicillin/sulbactam + probenicid, cefuroxine axetil + probenicid
Nocardia asteroides	Sulfonamides (high dose), trimethoprim/ sulfamethoxazole	Minocycline	Amikacin + imipenem + cefotaxime
Proteus mirabilis	Ampicillin	Trimethoprim/ sulphamethoxazole	
Proteus vulgaris	Parenteral 3rd general cephalosporin or fluoroquinolones	Antipseudomonal aminoglycoside	Imipenem, aztreonam
Pseudomonas aeruginosa	Parenteral 3rd generation antipseudomonal cephalosporin, imipenem, tobramycin	Fluoroquinolones, ticarcillin clavulanate, aztreonam	In some areas where tobramycin resistance is prevalent, amikacin is the choice
Salmonella typhi	Ciprofloxacin, ceftriaxone, cefoperazone, trimethoprim/ sulphamethoxazole	Chloramphenicol, ampicillin	Multidrug resistant strains common in many developing countries; seen in immigrants
Serratia marcescens	Gentamicin, parenteral 3rd generation cephalosporin, imipenem, fluoroquinolones	Aztreonam	
Staphylococcus aureus, methicillin sensitive	Penicillinase resistant synthetic penicillin	Vancomycin, erythromycin, clindamycin, parenteral 1st generation cephalosporin	Imipenem, amoxicillin clavulanate, ticarcillin clavulanate, ampicillin sulbactam
Staphylococcus aureus, methicillin resistant	Vancomycin	Teicoplanin	Fusidic acid; ciprofloxacin resistance in 80% of nosocomial infections
Staphylococcus epidermidis	Vancomycin		Penicillinase resistant synthetic penicillin or cephalothin

(contd)

Table 5.2 Antimicrobial agents of choice against selected organisms (contd)

Bacterial species	Recommended	Alternative	Also effective (comments)
Streptococcus, anaerobic (*Peptostreptococcus*)	Penicillin G	Clindamycin	Erythromycin, doxycycline, vancomycin
Streptococcus pneumoniae, penicillin sensitive	Penicillin G	Erythromycin, clindamycin	
Streptococcus pneumoniae, penicillin resistant	Vancomycin	Parenteral 3rd generation cephalosporin	Rifampin effective but resistance to appears rapidly
Streptococcus pyogenes, group A	Penicillin G or V	All β-lactams, erythromycin	

Documentation of systemic antibiotic levels

The concentration of drug must be high enough at the site of the infection to inhibit or, ideally, to kill the pathogens. At the same time the concentration of drug in the serum must be below levels which are toxic to the patient. Systemic levels of potentially toxic antibiotics are monitored by determining "peak" and "trough" concentrations. Peak concentrations are determined from peripheral blood obtained 30 minutes after administration of an intravenous antibiotic, and are adjusted by changing the amount of drug administered. Trough levels are determined from peripheral blood obtained just prior to antibiotic administration, and are adjusted by increasing or decreasing the interval of time between doses. The trough level of antibiotic in the serum should be four times the mean inhibitory concentration (MIC) of the antibiotic as determined for the specific pathogenic bacteria. If this is possible, the pathogen is considered to be sensitive. If it is not possible it is resistant.

Occasionally "tolerant" pathogens are encountered. Tolerance is defined as occurring when the mean bacteriocidal concentration is at least 32 times higher than the MIC (ie, the microorganism is inhibited but not killed by a given concentration of antibiotic). Although the significance of tolerance is still controversial, there is one study which indicates that it can be of clinical importance in vertebral osteomyelitis.[2]

Aminoglycosides and vancomycin must be carefully monitored to maintain their levels within the therapeutic range and below the levels which are toxic to the patient. These antibiotics are excreted by the kidney and have renal toxicity. Therefore, initial subclinical toxicity can result in increasing levels of antibiotic and significant toxicity. Peaks and troughs of potentially toxic antibiotics are monitored weekly. The penicillins, cephalosporins, clindamycin, and quinolones usually do not require determination of peaks and troughs, as they are not toxic. However, a CBC, albumin, BUN, and creatinine are obtained weekly to monitor bone marrow suppression, and liver and kidney toxicity.

Duration of systemic antibiotic therapy

The ideal duration of systemic antibiotic therapy is controversial. The rule of thumb based upon clinical studies has been four to six weeks.[3] As the duration of therapy increases so do the number of side effects, toxicity, and cost. On the other hand, it is possible that the longer a patient receives antibiotic the better the chance of long term suppression of infection. It is important to administer antibiotics in conjunction with appropriate surgery. If the surgery has been successful in eradicating all necrotic tissue, and, in effect, has converted an infected focus to a contaminated wound, Cierny and Mader postulate that the duration of antibiotic therapy can be shortened to three weeks.[4] This is the time necessary for granulation tissue to cover and protect débrided bone.

Technique: systemic antibiotic therapy

In most cases, antibiotics are initiated during the surgical débridement, after material for culture has been obtained. Antibiotic selection is based upon cultures of material obtained by swabbing the sinus tract or by biopsy. The operative cultures are considered definitive and the final antibiotic selection is based upon them. In cases in which venous access is a potential problem, either because of an absence of peripheral veins or because vancomycin or oxacillin will be administered, a central line is inserted. Antibiotics are administered for four to eight weeks, according to the clinical course. Peak and troughs are obtained at weekly intervals when potentially toxic antibiotics are administered. At the conclusion of therapy the central line is left in place for one to four weeks, so that if the patient has a recurrence of the infection it does not have to be reinserted.

Antibiotic therapy – local

There are three methods of local antibiotic delivery in use today: depot administration using PMMA-antibiotic composites; depot administration using biodegradable antibiotic composites; and local delivery with a pump. To describe each of these methods adequately, it is important to understand the general principles and history of local antibiotic therapy.

General principles of local antibiotic therapy

Bone and joint infections are localized infections and, therefore, are tailored for local antibiotic administration. Local antibiotic therapy has the potential for reducing the morbidity associated with prolonged systemic antibiotic administration. For local antibiotic therapy to be successful, the infected area must be managed with appropriate surgical procedures, the pathogenic organisms must be sensitive to the antibiotic being used, and the antibiotic must reach the entire infected area. One of the major risks of local antibiotic therapy is superinfection with aggressive panresistant organisms. Closed antibiotic delivery systems (ie, implanted PMMA–antibiotic beads) have less of a chance to become infected with resistant organisms, and thus have an advantage over open systems (ie, suction irrigation systems).

Historically, several methods of local antibiotic therapy have been attempted. Grace and Bryson were the first to describe irrigation as a method of delivering antibiotics locally.[5] Compere modified and popularized this technique.[6] Following débridement, the wound was closed over perforated inflow and outflow tubes. A solution consisting of detergent and novobiocin entered the wound via the inflow tube and was sucked out through the outflow tube. Systemic oral antibiotic administration was continued during local therapy. The problem with this method was superinfection with resistant organisms, in particular *Pseudomonas* and *Candida*. These organisms were exposed to the high local levels of antibiotic at the drainage tube sites and frequently invaded the wound.

Organ described arterial perfusion and Finsterbush and Weinberg described venous perfusion for chronic osteomyelitis.[7,8] Using these techniques, the extremity was isolated with a tourniquet and massive doses of antibiotic were injected intraarterially or intravenously. Problems with this method included the complicated nature of the technique and the limited duration of antibiotic therapy.

A number of European surgeons have investigated depot administration of antibiotics; ie, mixing antibiotics with a carrier, and depositing the resulting composite in the débrided wound. Many materials have been used as carriers: a blood coagulum; plaster of Paris; PMMA; and polylactic acid. In the 1950s, Winter and Bikfalvi and Ecke described depot administration of penicillin and streptomycin with autogenous coagulated blood in osteomyelitic defects.[9,10] Mackey et al studied in vitro elution of various antibiotics from plaster of Paris pellets.[11] They found that gentamicin had the most consistent elution properties, cefazolin and lincomycin eluted too quickly (no detectable levels by 20 and 5 days respectively). Plaster of Paris has the theoretical advantage that it is absorbed and a second operation would not be required; however, animal studies were not encouraging.[12] Buchholz described depot administration of antibiotics in PMMA in the management of infected total hips.[13,14] The method of local antibiotic delivery used most frequently today, PMMA-antibiotic beads, is a direct extension of this work. Hedstrom reported the injection of sinus tracts with dextran and cloxacillin, chloramphenicol or colistin.[15] This therapy was combined with appropriate systemic antibiotic therapy. Surgery was not performed and in many cases there were retained sequestra. As expected, there was a high percentage of recurrences. Becker and Spadaro reported the use of electrically generated silver ions in the treatment of orthopedic infections.[16] This was either in the form of a wire, or a silver nylon mesh packing

the wound. They felt treatment also stimulated bone formation at the anode. I have described local antibiotic administration via an implanted pump in the treatment of osteomyelitis and infected total joints.[17]

PMMA–antibiotic composites

The primary advantages of depot administration of antibiotic composites are that high local levels of antibiotic are achieved, and that the material from which the antibiotic leaches occupies the dead space created by débridement.

Following Buchholz's description of one stage revision arthroplasty with an antibiotic–PMMA composite, tremendous interest in PMMA as a carrier for antibiotics was generated.[13] Vecsei and Barquet reported their results using PMMA-gentamicin beads in the management of 25 patients with chronic osteomyelitis.[18] These 25 patients were selected from a group of 120. The authors credited Klemm as being the originator of the technique and described it as an alternative to suction drainage. Vecsei and Barquet attempted to close all wounds primarily. When primary closure was not possible a plastic film was applied to seal the wound. Intravenous antibiotics were administered in the perioperative period. In some cases the beads were replaced with autogenous cancellous graft; in others the beads were simply removed. The results were excellent, with long term suppression of infection in 22 of the 25 patients. While it is extremely difficult to interpret these results in the light of the variability of the management protocol and the selectivity of the series, two concepts are clear: the beads are useful to occupy dead space; and the beads serve as a local antibiotic delivery system.

Following the landmark studies of Buchholz and Vecsei and Barquet, a number of investigators studied the process of antibiotic elution from PMMA in depth. Wahlig et al studied patients who had undergone total hip arthroplasty with

PMMA–gentamicin composites.[19] They found that gentamicin levels in wound drainage fluid from around the prosthesis averaged 48 µg/ml in the first day and 12 µg/ml the second day. They calculated that roughly 7% of the gentamicin eventually eluted from the cement. This study highlights one of the basic problems of depot administration: that elution is limited and local antibiotic levels drop rapidly. Hill et al studied elution of various antibiotics from various types of cement.[20] They found that all tested antibiotics (gentamicin, fucidine, clindamycin, penicillin G, cephalothin, erythromycin, and colistin) maintained their biologic activity, and eluted from cement in large amounts in the first two to three days, after which there was a low concentration in the surrounding fluid. Prior to the study it was conjectured that heat labile antibiotics were inactivated by the heat of polymerization of the PMMA. Schurman et al found that the amount and rate of antibiotic eluting from PMMA was proportional to the surface area of the cement.[21] Hoff et al found that the concentration of antibiotics was higher at the bone–cement interface than areas further removed.[22] Elson et al reported that antibiotics eluted from Palacos R cement better than simplex, CMW and Sulfix cement.[23] Marks et al found that hardened PMMA was not significantly weakened by the addition of antibiotics.[24] This study laid to rest the concerns that early mechanical failure of revision arthroplasties would result from the addition of antibiotic to cement. Eckman et al described the "bead pouch technique" and advocated its use in the management of open fractures.[25] This technique consists of débridement, fracture stabilization, and packing the wound with PMMA–antibiotic beads. Wounds are closed primarily over a drain, or covered with an impermeable membrane. After the wound stabilizes, the beads are removed and a primary or secondary closure is performed. Minor hypersensitivity reactions to antibiotics delivered via PMMA have been reported; however, I have not found a single report of major allergic reaction.[26]

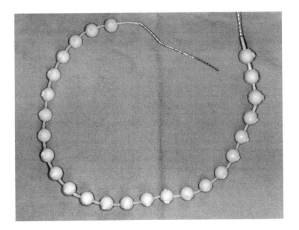

Figure 5.1

PMMA–antibiotic beads.

Technique: PMMA–antibiotic composites

The PMMA–antibiotic beads are available from the pharmacy in many hospitals (Fig 5.1). When they are not available from the pharmacy, beads are made by mixing powdered antibiotics with PMMA polymer. Prior to adding the liquid monomer, the antibiotic must be well dispersed in the polymer, or elution will be unpredictable and may be decreased. The antibiotic and powdered cement are stirred until there is no doubt that they are well mixed. Alternatively, a small amount of a sterile powdered dye can be added. When the powdered dye is well dispersed, the antibiotic is assumed to also be dispersed. Vancomycin is unique in that it forms aggregates which must be powdered prior to mixing. Virtually any powdered antibiotic can be added to cement. Commonly used antibiotics and amounts per 40 g pack of cement are: cephazolin, 1 or 2 g; vancomycin 1 or 2 g, and tobramycin 1.2 to 3.6 g. After the polymer and the antibiotic have been mixed, the liquid monomer is added. As the volume of antibiotic is increased per given amount of cement, the time of polymerization of the cement increases. When the PMMA–

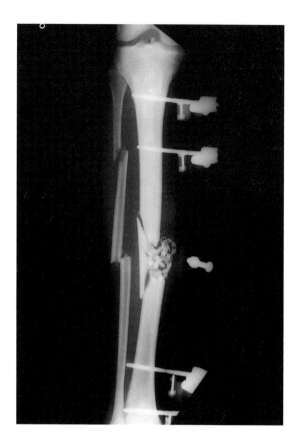

Figure 5.2

Radiograph of a tibia in which a defect has been filled with PMMA–antibiotic beads.

antibiotic composite has reached the stage that it is workable, and does not readily adhere to surgical gloves, it is rolled into small balls and strung on heavy nonabsorbable suture. After polymerization is completed, and the composite has cooled, the beads are implanted in the defect. Care is taken to fill the defect as completely as possible, leaving the minimum amount of dead space unoccupied (Fig 5.2). Following implantation of beads, the wound is always closed, to prevent the emergence of bacterial strains that are resistant to the antibiotics in the beads.

The timing of bead removal is determined by the rate and amount of antibiotic elution and the fact that after three to four weeks the beads become progressively entrapped in scar tissue and removal becomes more and more difficult. We usually remove beads three to six weeks after they are implanted. Following bead removal, the defect which they occupied is reconstructed, most frequently with autogenous cancellous bone graft or a soft tissue transfer.

Biodegradable carriers

The primary disadvantage of PMMA as an antibiotic carrier is that it must be removed. Removal of beads usually requires a surgical procedure and creates dead space which must be addressed. These disadvantages have generated interest in developing an absorbable carrying material for depot administration of antibiotics. Setterstrom et al developed the concept of encapsulating antibiotics in microspheres for topical administration.[27] Jacob et al reported the use of encapsulated microspheres of antibiotic in the prevention of infection in a rabbit open tibia fracture model.[28,29] These investigators found: high local levels and low systemic levels of antibiotic; and a low incidence of infection in rabbits treated with antibiotic encapsulated microspheres. The primary drawback to antibiotic encapsulated microspheres is that dead space is not addressed. An alternative to antibiotic microspheres is blocks of bioabsorbable or bioerodeable material impregnated with antibiotics (Fig 5.3). Laurencin et al studied the release of gentamicin from blocks of polyanhydride in a rat osteomyelitis model.[30] They found lower bacterial counts in rats treated with the polyanhydride-gentamicin composite than in animals without an implant or treated with a PMMA–gentamicin implant. Wei et al studied the release of antibiotic from polylactic acid blocks.[31] Gerhart et al and Nelson et al have studied the release of various antibiotics from polyanhydrides.[32,33] Gerhart et al compared the release of gentamicin and vancomycin from a biodegradable bone cement

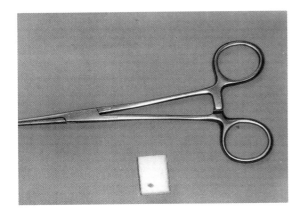

Figure 5.3

Polylactic acid block.

(polypropylene fumarate-methylmethacrylate) with release from PMMA.[32] They found that, over a 14 day period, local antibiotic levels were significantly higher around the biodegrad-

able bone cement. Local vancomycin levels around the biodegradable bone cement were 20 times greater than levels around the PMMA. Shinto et al found that gentamicin, cefoperazone and flomoxef were released in a controlled fashion from bioabsorbable calcium hydroxyapatite ceramic blocks.[34] The techniques of local delivery of antibiotics via biodegradable carriers are evolving, and have not yet been standardized; therefore, they are not included in this chapter.

Implanted pump

I developed an alternative method of local antibiotic delivery using an implantable pump.[18,35,36] This system is completely closed and thus decreases the incidence of superinfection. The pump (Figs 5.4, 5.5) (Shiley Infusaid, Norwood, MA, USA) consists of two chambers separated by collapsible titanium bellows. One chamber of the bellows is filled with drug. The

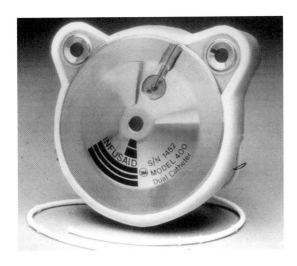

Figure 5.4

The implantable drug pump used to deliver antibiotics locally in the treatment of orthopedic infections.

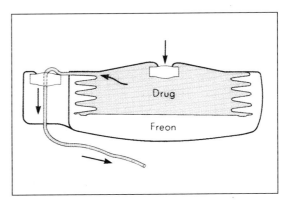

Figure 5.5

Schematic drawing of the implantable drug pump. The pump is divided into two chambers by flexible titanium bellows. One chamber is filled with drug. The second is filled with a charging fluid. As the charging fluid expands it compresses the drug chamber, driving the drug out of the outflow catheter.

other chamber is filled with freon. As the freon expands it compresses the drug chamber, forcing the drug out through the outflow catheter. The pump holds 50 ml of drug and delivers 5–7 ml of drug per 24 hours. The pump is refilled percutaneously through the inlet septum at weekly intervals, reexpanding the drug chamber and driving the freon back into its liquid phase. Local antibiotic delivery via an implantable pump can be used with other techniques in the management of bone and joint infections. Its use does not preclude PMMA–antibiotic beads, or small wire circular frame external fixaters.

The drug most frequently used in the pump is amikacin, at a concentration of 50 mg/ml. Amikacin is used for three reasons. (1) Amikacin is an aminoglycoside. Like other aminoglycosides (gentamicin, tobramycin, and netilmicin) it is stable in the pump. Other drugs, such as the cephalosporins and vancomycin, are not.[37] (2) Amikacin induces tolerance in bacteria at a lower rate than other aminoglycosides.[38] (3) Amikacin is a bactericidal drug with a broad spectrum of activity, which includes *Staphylococcus aureus* and Gram negative bacilli.[38,39] There are three disadvantages of using amikacin. (1) Amikacin has significant eighth nerve toxicity and nephrotoxicity when administered systemically. However, with an implantable pump, between 250 mg and 350 mg of amikacin is delivered per day. This is one third the recommended systemic dose; therefore, systemic toxicity is seldom a problem. (2) Amikacin is not effective against *Candida* or anaerobes; therefore, patients with infections caused by these organisms cannot be treated with this method. In addition, the patient is at risk for a superinfection with *Candida*. (3) *Enterococcus* is resistant to amikacin; however it is sensitive to the combination of amikacin and ampicillin. If *Enterococcus* is the pathogen, ampicillin is administered intravenously in the perioperative period, and orally during the remainder of therapy.

The complications unique to local antibiotic delivery via an implantable pump are: pump or catheter infection; displacement of the pump; and migration of the outflow catheters. Approximately 10% of patients developed pump site or catheter infection. When this occurs, it often responds to oral administration of the appropriate antibiotic. If only the catheter is involved it can be revised. All patients in whom the pump site or catheters have become infected have responded to removal of the pump, closure over a drain, and a short course of systemic antibiotics (7–14 days). There have been no lasting pump site infections and no surgeries necessary following pump removal. Since 1992 we have perforated one of the outflow catheters with a suture as it leaves the pump. This results in some antibiotic being delivered to the pump pocket and has decreased the incidence of pump site infection. In approximately 1.5% of cases the pump has flipped or rotated. In these cases the pump site was opened, the pump was repositioned and firmly sutured to the fascia. In 1% of cases (2 patients) the catheters have migrated from the infected area. Both cases involved infected joints – an elbow and a knee. In both cases the catheter had been sutured to soft tissue in the infected area. Why it continued to pull out is not clear.

Technique: local antibiotic delivery via an implanted pump for osteomyelitis

Precautions are taken to protect the pump site from becoming infected. The pump site and infected area are prepped using two separate surgical scrubs, taking care not to cross-contaminate the pump site with soap from the infected area. During pump implantation the infected area is covered with an impermeable drape. The pump is implanted through a transverse incision made at the level of the umbilicus. A pocket is formed superficial to the preabdominal fascia and the pump is sutured to the fascia. Meticulous hemostasis is maintained at the pump site, as a postoperative hematoma could become infected. The outflow catheters are led distally towards the infected area. They are brought through the skin, coiled, and held in place with an adhesive drape. After the pump site is closed, both it and the catheters are covered with a sterile impermeable drape to prevent contamination during the management of the infected area. After the infected area has been managed surgically, the outflow catheters are brought distally and placed in the wound to achieve the best spread of antibiotic. The catheters are sutured into place using fine absorbable suture, and the wound is closed. In most cases a suction drain is left in the wound.

Postoperatively, serum amikacin levels and local levels from the wound drainage are monitored. A minimum of five doses of systemic antibiotics are administered to protect the pump site and to treat the cellulitis frequently associated with bone and joint infections. The patient is carefully observed for signs of infection at the pump site. The pump is refilled at weekly intervals. Pump removal is based on the clinical course and how well the pump is tolerated. We leave the pump in for a minimum of six weeks. Pump removal is an outpatient procedure. Usually the outflow catheters come out easily with the pump. If the catheters break, we leave them when there are no signs or symptoms of infection. If the patient is still actively infected, broken catheters must be removed so that they do not act as a residual nidus of infection.

Technique: local antibiotic delivery via an implanted pump for infected arthroplasties

Infected arthroplasties are managed somewhat differently than osteomyelitis. We divide infected arthroplasties into two groups: septic arthritis; and infections involving the bone–prosthesis interface (BPI). The distinction is made on clinical and radiographic bases. A history of previous surgery involving the infected joint and duration of symptoms for more than six weeks indicate probable involvement of the BPI. Radiographic signs of loosening or radiolucent defects at the BPI indicate involvement. In patients with septic arthritis (the BPI is not infected) the pump is

implanted, and the joint is exposed through the previous incision and irrigated thoroughly. A synovectomy is not performed, the prosthesis is left in situ, the outflow catheters are sutured in the joint, and the joint is closed over drains. The drains are left in place until there is less than 10 ml of drainage per 8 hours (usually 3–7 days). Postoperatively, the extremity is placed on a continuous passive motion machine.

In cases in which the BPI is involved, a two stage revision is performed. The pump is implanted as described. All components, cement, necrotic bone, and infected soft tissue are removed. The resulting dead space is packed with PMMA–antibiotic beads in infected hip arthroplasties or a PMMA–antibiotic block in infected knee arthroplasties. The outflow catheters from the pump are placed in the wound and the wound is closed over drains. Postoperatively, patients with chronically infected total hip arthroplasties are placed in balanced skeletal traction. Patients with chronically infected total knee arthroplasties have the involved extremity placed in a compression dressing and knee immobilizer. The drains are discontinued when drainage is less than 10 ml per 8 hours. Based on the clinical appearance of the wound, a revision arthroplasty is performed four to eight weeks after the initial surgery. At the time of revision, the beads or spacer are removed and a prosthesis is cemented into place using a PMMA–antibiotic composite. The outflow catheters from the pump are left in the joint. Suction drains and continuous passive motion are used postoperatively.

Maximizing the physiologic status of the patient

In most cases the physiologic status of the patient is stable. However, stability is not the rule and occasionally a patient with a bone and joint infection will present in septic shock, and require immediate support. This is most likely to occur in toxic shock syndrome, tetanus, gas gangrene, necrotizing fasciitis, and overwhelming septicemia. The general rules of management are: remove the focus of infection (frequently requires amputation); aggressive fluid replacement (requires a central line or Swann–Ganz catheter to monitor central pressure); and antibiotic administration (to sterilize the focus of infection). In addition, there must be the capability to diagnose and manage: potential renal failure; adult respiratory distress syndrome; loss of airway; disseminated intravascular coagulation; and cardiac arrhythmias.

In most cases the physiologic status of the patient is not an immediate threat. Nevertheless, improving the physiologic status will decrease the incidence of complications and increase the incidence of success. The two most frequently encountered detriments are smoking and malnutrition. Smoking clearly affects the rate of complications after free tissue transfers, and slows consolidation of regenerated bone, increasing the duration of disability when small wire circular fixaters are utilized. The patient should be willing to quit smoking several months prior to reconstructive procedures.

Malnutrition

Malnutrition is not as obvious as smoking, but is equally detrimental to the clinical course. The incidence of malnutrition in the hospital population has been estimated to be 50%.[40] Protein calorie malnutrition is associated with increased postoperative morbidity and mortality.[41–44] Overall protein depletion is associated with poor wound healing. Diminished levels of visceral protein are directly related to reduced immunocompetency. Einhorn et al showed that protein and mineral malnutrition induced in rats immediately after a creation of an experimental femur fracture did not decrease the early healing potential.[45] However, the fracture callus never achieved normal strength. The authors speculate that the rat was able to mobilize stores of protein and minerals from other sites, but that once these stores were depleted the ability to heal was diminished.

The management of malnutrition has two phases: identification of clinically relevant deficiencies; and correction of the deficiencies. The three methods used to assess nutritional deficiencies are: anthropometric, or somatic, measurements; laboratory tests; and a history and physical examination. Anthropometric measurements include: height and weight; arm circumference, which reflects muscle mass; and triceps skinfold thickness (measured with a caliper), which reflects subcutaneous fat. Laboratory tests include: the measurement of the serum proteins albumin and transferrin, both of which reflect visceral protein; the absolute lymphocyte count (the percentage of lymphocytes in the differential multiplied by the total white blood cell count); and skin reactivity. Dickhaut et al and Pinzur et al studied the relationship between wound healing and laboratory parameters.[46,47] Dickhaut et al found that Syme's amputations healed in 86% of diabetic patients with a serum albumin over 3.5 g/dl, and a total lymphocyte count of 1500/ml.[46] Patients with albumin and lymphocyte counts below these levels healed a Syme's amputation only 19% of the time. Pinzur et al reported similar results in a series of 64 patients undergoing a midfoot amputation.[47] They studied three parameters: the ankle arm index; the total lymphocyte count, and the serum albumin level. They found that when the ankle arm index, total lymphocyte count and serum albumin were above minimum levels, the rate of healing increased. The total lymphocyte count and the serum albumin were prospectively increased by means of hyperalimentation (usually oral) to 1500 cells/ml and to 3.0 g/dl, respectively, in 12 patients. Incisions in 11 of these 12 patients healed uneventfully.

A pertinent history includes determining whether there has been: weight loss; edema; anorexia; vomiting; diarrhea; decreased or unusual food intake; and chronic disease. The physical examination identifies jaundice, cheilosis, glossitis, muscle wasting, and edema. Baker et al found that a carefully taken history was reproducible and as accurate in assessing the nutritional status as various anthropometric measurements and laboratory values.[48]

Investigators have combined laboratory and anthropometric measurements in an attempt to predict the incidence of complications more accurately. Bistrian et al originated the "creatinine height index".[49] This value is determined by dividing the amount of creatinine actually excreted in a 24 hour period by the expected amount. The expected amount is based on the patient's height and correlates with muscle mass and thus protein reserves. Patients with malnutrition have decreased protein reserves and thus a decrease in the amount of creatinine actually excreted. In these patients the creatinine index is less than one. Dempsey et al developed a prognostic nutritional index (PNI) by prospectively recording various nutritional parameters in preoperative patients.[50] Using regression analysis, these parameters were then correlated with the incidence of complications following surgery. From this process the following formula evolved:

$$PNI(\%) = 158 - 16.6(Alb) - 0.78(TSF)$$
$$- 0.20(TFN) - 5.8(DH)$$

where Alb is the serum albumin concentration, TSF is the triceps skin fold, TFN is the serum transferrin concentration, and DH is skin test reactivity to any antigen to which the patient has been exposed (usually *Candida*): 0 is nonreactive, 1 is less than 5 mm, 2 is greater than 5 mm. Dempsey found that 87% of patients with postoperative complications and 96% of postoperative deaths were in patients with a PNI of greater than 50%.

Technique: maximization of physiologic status

Patients undergoing elective surgery for bone and joint infections are carefully examined and a detailed history is obtained at the initial visit. As part of the examination, the patient is examined for jaundice, muscle wasting, peripheral edema, and ascites. These are all indicators that the patient may be malnourished. Likewise, a history detailing the patient's eating habits, whether he or she is a smoker, and whether there has been loss of appetite, vomiting or diarrhea is obtained. I limit the laboratory workup for malnutrition to the serum albumin and total lymphocyte count. These should be above 3.5 mg/ml and 1500 cells/ml respectively. If the physical examination, history, or laboratory values indicate malnutrition, a nutritional consult is obtained and surgery is postponed until the serum albumin is above 3.5 mg/ml and the total lymphocyte count is above 1500. Usually nutritional deficiencies can be corrected by supplementing the diet orally, but occasionally enteral or even hyperalimentation is required. In addition, patients who smoke are asked to quit.

Electrical and magnetic fields

Wolff's law, stated over 100 years ago, is that bone grows and remodels in response to mechanical stresses. Fukada and Yasuda were the first to demonstrate that, when stressed, bone produces small electrical potentials due to minute spatial changes in the crystalline structure of the bone matrix and hydroxyapatite.[51] Compression results in a negative charge, while tension results in a positive charge. Fukada and Yasuda surmised that these piezoelectric potentials might act as the signal which directs bone growth and remodeling.

Anderson and Erikson found that "streaming potentials" occur in bone when it is deformed.[52] Streaming potentials have since been identified as a major source of mechanically generated electrical potentials. Streaming potentials occur because of a difference in electrical charges of the relatively free flowing interstitial fluid and the stationary bone matrix and hydroxyapatite crystals. When stressed, the bone deforms and changes shape. This displaces the interstitial fluid, and separates charged ions in the fluid from those fixed to the bone matrix and hydroxyapatite crystals. The separation of charge results in electrical potentials, termed streaming potentials.

That electrical potentials direct bone growth and remodeling is not in doubt. That electrical potentials some how also direct healing of fractures and consolidation of nonunions has its basis in work reported by Becker and later by Friedenberg and Brighton.[53,54] These investigators showed that the site of injury or fracture has a negative electrical charge and that altering the electrical potential also alters the progression of healing. The culmination of this experimental work was the clinical use of electrical fields to induce healing of nonunions and delayed unions.

The three types of electrical stimulation used to induce bone healing are: direct current; inductive coupling; and capacitive coupling. The mechanism of action of electrical fields is not known, and the mechanisms which apply to direct current stimulation probably differs from those driving stimulation by inductive and capacitive coupling.[55] Direct current is known to affect the local environment of the nonunion. Around the cathode there is a decrease in the partial pressure of oxygen and an increase in the pH.[56] Both of these changes favor bone formation. Whether this is the only mechanism at work in direct current stimulation is not known. Mechanisms of action of inductive and capacitive coupling are even less clear. One theory is that the electrical signal is a "first messenger" which induces differentiation of primitive stem cells to osteoblasts by altering ion permeability of the cell membrane.

Contraindications to all three types of electrical stimulation are: unacceptable malalignment;

the presence of a synovial pseudoarthrosis; and a gap greater than half the diameter of the bone.[57] Direct current is contraindicated in cases in which there is active infection. When implantation of the electrodes has activated a latent infection, direct current electrical stimulation is discontinued and the electrodes are removed.

Direct current

Direct current is applied via electrodes implanted in the area to be stimulated. The most frequently used direct current stimulator is totally implanted. This requires a surgical procedure, and is the primary disadvantage of this mode of electrical stimulation. On the other hand, once implanted, the device functions independently. Jorgenson reported a selected series of 28 nonunions of the tibia, forearm, humerus, and femur managed with direct current.[58] Many of these nonunions were infected, and Jorgenson emphasized that "all osteosynthesis material and any sequestra are removed". In all cases an external fixater was applied to stabilize the nonunion and direct current was applied through the external fixater pins. In some cases the nonunion was bone grafted. All 28 nonunions consolidated, after 1.5–10.0 months of stimulation. While it is difficult to interpret the results of this study, it is clear that direct current is an effective adjunct in the management of nonunions. A more accurate reflection of the incidence of success using direct current alone in the management of nonunions is found in a series reported by Day.[59] She managed 16 patients with nonunion of the tibia, femur, or upper extremity with direct current and casting. Eleven nonunions consolidated.

Inductive coupling

Inductive coupling consists of applying a magnetic field across the area to be stimulated by means of external coils. The magnetic field induces an electrical field in the tissues between the coils. Inductive coupling is often referred to as pulsed electromagnetic fields (PEMFs). This method is exacting, in that the patient is required to wear the coils eight hours a day and that the precise position of the coils and space between the coils is important: Sharrard reported a double blind study in which 45 patients with delayed union of the tibia were managed with PEMF or a placebo.[60] At 12 weeks 9 of 20 delayed unions in the PEMF group had healed, while only one of 25 delayed unions in the placebo group had healed. Although there has been controversy as to who had control of the randomization code during the study (Sharrard), I am convinced that this study proves that PEMFs induce consolidation of delayed unions of the tibia, even when applied only for 12 weeks.[61]

Recently, a new type of inductive coupling stimulator has become available. This stimulator produces very low amplitude magnetic fields. The fields are referred to as combined low energy magnetic fields (CLEMFs). CLEMFs are applied only one hour per day, and the coil position is not as precise as that required for PEMF. OrthoLogic, Phoenix, Arizona, USA, supplies CLEMF devices, while EBI, Parsippany, New Jersey, USA, supplies PEMF devices.

Capacitive coupling

Capacitive coupling is achieved by applying capacitor plates to the area to be stimulated. As the plates become charged they induce an electrical field in the target tissues. Capacitive coupling is not as exacting a technique as PEMF. The management of nonunions with capacitively coupled electrical fields was reported by Brighton and Pollack.[62] Their series included 22 patients with nonunions. Overall, the success rate was 77%. Among these 22 patients were four patients with latent osteomyelitis, ie, no drainage at the time of management. All four had nonunions of the tibia. Of these four, only one patient failed to heal and he did not follow

the protocol. The authors conclude that osteomyelitis is not a contraindication for electrical stimulation.

Technique: electrical stimulation of nonunions

In cases in which the nonunion or delayed union is in acceptable alignment, CLEMFs are used, regardless of whether infection is present. If there are no signs of consolidation by four months, electrical stimulation is discontinued. Patient activity is based upon the patient's tolerance and the type of fixation (eg, a plated tibia is nonweight bearing).

Hyperbaric oxygen

Hyperbaric oxygen is directed at the local hypovascularity and hypoxia associated with chronic bone and joint infections. When a patient breathes 100% oxygen at 2.5 atmospheres, hemoglobin becomes saturated, and an additional 5.2 volume % dissolves in the plasma, resulting in a 20-fold increase in the oxygen diffusion gradient between the blood and avascular tissue. This gradient results in a marked increase of oxygenation of avascular areas. The increased oxygenation is effective because: it is directly bactericidal; it enhances the oxidative killing of bacteria by leukocytes; and it induces capillary angiogenesis, thus resulting in permanent improvement of local vascularity.[63] Theoretically, these factors make hyperbaric oxygen a potentially powerful adjuvant in the management of infections associated with local hypovascularity due to radionecrosis, diabetes, and chronic infection. Conversely, hyperbaric oxygen is of no value in the management of well perfused wounds.

Hyperbaric oxygen is clearly an effective adjunct in the management of clostridial myonecrosis. However, the use of hyperbaric oxygen in the management of bone and joint infections is controversial, because it is administered in conjunction with surgical management (ie, débridement and soft tissue coverage) and antibiotic therapy. Support for hyperbaric oxygen as an effective adjuvant in the management of chronic osteomyelitis is found in studies reported by Morrey et al and Davis et al.[64,65] In both studies, patients with posttraumatic or postsurgical chronic osteomyelitis were managed with surgical débridement and systemic antibiotic administration. Therapy was successful in 85–90% of cases, although in both reports the authors acknowledge that recurrence was a possibility. Neither of these studies is definitive, as they lack control subjects who were treated with surgical débridement and antibiotics, but who did not receive hyperbaric oxygen.

Technique: hyperbaric oxygen

Administration of hyperbaric oxygen requires access to a chamber and trained technicians. Hyperbaric oxygen is administered for 1–14 weeks in daily or twice daily treatments lasting approximately 90 minutes. The patient is placed in a chamber in which the pressure is increased to 2.4–3.0 atmospheres. One hundred per cent oxygen is then pumped into the chamber.

References

1   Wenger DR, Bobechko WP, Gilday DL, The spectrum of intervertebral disc-space infection in children, *J Bone Joint Surg* (1978) **60A**:100–108.

2   Musher DM, Fletcher T, Tolerant *Staphylococcus aureus* causing vertebral osteomyelitis, *Arch Intern Med* (1982) **142**:631.

3   Waldvogel FA, Medoff G, Swartz MD, Osteomyelitis: a review of clinical features, therapeutic considerations and unusual aspects, *N Engl J Med* (1970) **282**:198.

4   Cierny G, Mader JT, Adult chronic osteomyelitis, *Orthopedics* (1984) **7**:1557.

5   Grace EJ, Bryson V, Topical use of concentrated penicillin in surface-active solution, *Arch Surg* (1945) **50**:219–222.

6   Compere EL, Treatment of osteomyelitis and infected wounds by closed irrigation with a detergent-antibiotic solution, *Acta Orthop Scand* (1962) **32**:324–333.

7   Organ CH Jr, The utilization of massive doses of antimicrobial agents with isolation perfusion in the treatment of chronic osteomyelitis: intermediate term results, *Clin Orthop Rel Res* (1971) **76**:185–193.

8   Finsterbush A, Weinberg H, Venous perfusion of the limb with antibiotics for osteomyelitis and other chronic infections, *J Bone Joint Surg* (1972) **54A**:1227–1234.

9   Winter L, Management of chronic osteitis and osteomyelitis with a coagulum of autogenous blood + penicillin + thrombin, on the base of 56 case reports, *J Int Chir* (1951) **11**:510–524.

10   Bikfalvi A, Ecke H, Die behandlung der chronischen osteomyelitis mit der eigenblut-antibiotika-plombe, *Bruns Beitr Klin Chir* (1960) **201**:190–207.

11   Mackey D, Varlet A, Debeaumont D, Antibiotic loaded plaster of paris pellets: an *in-vitro* study of a possible method of local antibiotic therapy in bone infection, *Clin Orthop Rel Res* (1982) **167**:263–268.

12   Dahners LE, Funderburk CH, Gentamicin loaded plaster of paris as a treatment of experimental osteomyelitis in rabbits, *Clin Orth Rel Res* (1987) **219**:278–282.

13 Buchholz HW, Gartmann HD, Infektions – prophylaxe und operative Behandlung der schleichenden tiefen infektion bei der totalen endoprosthese, *Chirurg* (1972) **43**:446.

14 Buchholz LS, Elson RA, Heniert K, Antibiotic-loaded acrylic cement: current concepts, *Clin Orthop* (1984) **190**:96.

15 Hedstrom SA, General and local antibiotic treatment of chronic osteomyelitis, *Scand J Infect Dis* (1969) **1**:175–180.

16 Becker RO, Spadaro JA, Treatment of orthopaedic infections with electrically generated silver ions. A preliminary report, *J Bone Joint Surg* (1978) **60A**:871–881.

17 Perry CR, Davenport K, Vossen MK, Local delivery of antibiotics via an implantable pump in the treatment of osteomyelitis, *Clin Orthop Rel Res* (1988) **226**:222.

18 Vecsei V, Barquet A, Treatment of chronic osteomyelitis by necrectomy and gentamicin-PMMA beads, *Clin Orthop Rel Res* (1981) **159**:201.

19 Wahlig H, Dingeldein E, Buchholz HW et al, Pharmacokinetic study of gentamicin-loaded cement in total hip replacements, comparative effects of varying dosage, *J Bone Joint Surg* (1984) **66B**:175–179.

20 Hill J, Klenerman L, Trustey S, et al, Diffusion of antibiotics from acrylic bone-cement *in-vitro*, *J Bone Joint Surg* (1977) **59B**:197–199.

21 Schurman DJ, Trindade C, Hirschman HP et al, Antibiotic-acrylic bone cement composites, studies of gentamicin and palacos, *J Bone Joint Surg* (1978) **60A**:978–984.

22 Hoff SF, Fitzgerald RH, Kelly PJ, The depot administration of penicillin G and gentamicin in acrylic bone cement, *J Bone Joint Surg* (1981) **63A**:798–804.

23 Elson RA, Jephcott AE, McGechie BD, et al, Antibiotic-loaded acrylic cement, *J Bone Joint Surg* (1977) **59B**:200–205.

24 Marks KE, Nelson CL, Lautenschlager EP, Antibiotic-impregnated acrylic bone cement, *J Bone Joint Surg* (1976) **58A**:358–364.

25 Eckman JB, Henry SL, Mangino PD, et al, Wound and serum levels of tobramycin with prophylactic use of tobramycin-impregnated polymethylmethacrylate beads in compound fractures, *Clin Orthop Rel Res* (1988) **237**:213–215.

26 Scheife RT, Levy M, Greenblatt DJ, Antimicrobial agents. In: Miller RR, Greenblatt DJ, eds, *Drug effects in hospitalized patients: experiences of the Boston collaborative drug surveillance program 1966–1975* (New York: Wiley 1976): 242–245.

27 Setterstrom JA, Tice TR, Myers WE, Development of encapsulated antibiotics for topical administration to wounds. In: Kim SW, ed, *Recent advances in drug delivery systems* (Plenum: New York 1984) 185–198.

28 Jacob E, Setterstrom JA, Bach DE et al, Evaluation of biodegradable ampicillin amhydrate microcapsules for local treatment of exerimental staphylococcal osteomyelitis, *Clin Orthop Rel Res* (1991) **267**:237–244.

29 Jacob E, Cierny G III, Fallon MI et al, Evaluation of biodegradeable cefazolin sodium microspheres for the prevention of infection in rabbits with experimental open tibial fractures stabelized with internal fixation, *J Orthop Res* (1993) **11**:404–411.

30 Laurencin CT, Gerhart T, Witschger P et al, Bioerodible polyanhydrides for antibiotic drug delivery: in vivo osteomyelitis treatment in a rat model system, *J Orthop Res* (1993) **11**:256–262.

31 Wei G, Kotoura Y, Oka M et al, A bioabsorbable delivery system for antibiotic treatment of osteomyelitis, the use of lactic acid

oligomer as a carrier, *J Bone Joint Surg* (1991) **73B**:246–252.

32   Gerhart TN, Roux RD, Horowitz G, et al, Antibiotic release from an experimental biodegradable bone cement, *J Orthop Res* (1988) **6**:585–592.

33   Nelson CL, Hickmon SG, Skinner RA, Antibiotic levels produced in adjacent bone, wound exudate, serum, and urine by a biodegradable delivery system, *Trans Orthop Res Soc* (1992) **17**:431.

34   Shinto Y, Uchida A, Korkususz F et al, Calcium hydroxyapatite ceramic used as a delivery system for antibiotics, *J Bone Joint Surg* (1992) **74B**:600–604.

35   Perry CR, Rice S, Ritterbusch JK, et al, Local administration of antibiotics with an implantable osmotic pump, *Clin Orthop Rel Res* (1985) **182**:284.

36   Perry CR, Ritterbusch JK, Rice SH et al, Antibiotics delivered by an implantable drug pump: a new application for treating osteomyelitis, *Am J Med* (1986) **80**:222.

37   Perry CR, Ellington LL, Becker A et al, Antibiotic stability in an implantable pump, *J Orthop Res* (1986) **4**:494.

38   Rusticcia AM, Cunha BA, The aminoglycosides, *Med Clin North Am* (1982) **66**:303.

39   Aldridge KE, Janney A, Sanders CV, Comparison of the activities of coumermycin, ciprofloxacin, teicoplanin, and other non-B-lactam antibiotics against clinical isolates of methicillin-resistant *Staphylococcus aureus* from various geographical locations, *Antimicrob Agents and Chemother* (1985) **28**:634.

40   Bistrian BR, Blackburn GL, Vitale J, et al, Prevalence of malnutrition in general medical patients, *JAMA* (1976) **235**:1567–1570.

41   Mullen JL, Gertner MH, Buzby GP, et al, Implications of malnutrition in the surgical patient, *Arch Surg* (1979) **114**:121–125.

42   Reinhardt GF, Myscofski JW, Wilkens DB, et al, Incidence of mortality of hypoalbuminemic patients in hospitalized veterans, *J Parenter Enteral Nutr* (1980) **4**:357–359.

43   Patterson BM, Cornell CN, Carbone B, et al, Protein depletion and metabolic stress in elderly patients who have a fracture of the hip, *J Bone Joint Surg* (1992) **74A**:251–260.

44   Jensen JE, Jensen TG, Smith TK, et al, Nutrition in orthopedic surgery, *J Bone Joint Surg* (1982) **64A**:1263–1272.

45   Einhorn TA, Bonnarens F, Burstein AH, The contributions of dietary protein and mineral to the healing of experimental fractures. A biomechanical study, *J Bone Joint Surg* (1986) **68A**:1389–1395.

46   Dickhaut SC, DeLee JC, Page CP, Nutritional status: importance in predicting wound healing after amputation, *J Bone Joint Surg* (1984) **66A**:71–75.

47   Pinzur M, Kaminsky M, Sage R, et al, Amputations at the middle level of the foot. A retrospective and perspective review, *J Bone Joint Surg* (1986) **68A**:1061–1064.

48   Baker JP, Detsky AS, Wesson DE, et al, Nutritional assessment - a comparison of clinical judgement and objective measurements, *N Eng J Med* (1982) **36**:969–972.

49   Bistrian BR, Blackburn GL, Sherman M, et al, Therapeutic index of nutritional depletion in hospitalized patients, *Surg Gynecol Obstet* (1975) **141**:512–516.

50   Dempsey DT, Buzby GP, Mullen JL, Nutritional assessment in the seriously ill patient, *J Am Coll Nutr* (1983) **2**:15–23.

51 Fukada E, Yasuda I, On the piezoelectric effect of bone, *J Physiol Soc Japan* (1957) **12**:1158–1162.

52 Anderson JC, Erikson C, Piezoelectric properties of dry and wet bone, *Nature* (1970) **227**:491–492.

53 Becker RO, The bioelectric factors in amphibian limb regeneration, *J Bone Joint Surg* (1961) **43A**:643–656.

54 Friedenberg ZB, Brighton CT, Bioelectric potentials in bone, *J Bone Joint Surg* (1966) **48A**:915–923.

55 Lavine LS, Lustrin I, Shamos MH, Treatment of congenital pseudoarthrosis of the tibia with direct current, *Clin Orthop Rel Res* (1977) **124**:69–74.

56 Baranowski TJ, Black J, Brighton CT, Microenvironmental changes associated with electrical stimulation of osteogenesis by direct current, *J Electrochem Soc* (1983) **130**:120.

57 Connolly JF, Selection, evaluation and indications for electrical stimulation of ununited fractures, *Clin Orthop Rel Res* (1981) **161**:39–53.

58 Jorgenson TE, Asymmetrical slow-pulsing direct current, *Clin Orthop Rel Res* (1981) **161**:67–70.

59 Day L, Electrical stimulation in the treatment of ununited fractures, *Clin Orthop Rel Res* (1981) **161**:54–57.

60 Sharrard WJ, A double blind trial of pulsed electromagnetic fields for delayed union of tibial fractures, *J Bone Joint Surg* (1990) **72B**:347–355.

61 Sharrard WJ, Pulsed electromagnetic fields (letter), *J Bone Joint Surg* (1992) **74B**:630.

62 Brighton CT, Pollack SR, Treatment of recalcitrant non-union with a capacitively coupled electrical field. A preliminary report, *J Bone Joint Surg* (1985) **67A**:577–585.

63 Knighton DR, Oredson S, Banda M, et al, Regulation of repair: hypoxic control of macrophage mediated angiogenesis, In: Hunt TK, Heppenstall RB, Pines E, et al, eds, *Biological and clinical aspects of soft and hard tissue repair* (Praeger: New York) 41–49.

64 Morrey BF, Dunn JM, Heimbach RD, et al, Hyperbaric oxygen and chronic osteomyelitis, *Clin Orthop Rel Res* (1979) **144**:121–127.

65 Davis JC, Heckman JD, DeLee JC, et al, Chronic non-hematogenous osteomyelitis treated with adjuvant hyperbaric oxygen, *J Bone Joint Surg* (1986) **68A**:1210–1217.

6
OPERATIVE MANAGEMENT OF OSTEOMYELITIS

The surgical management of bone and joint infections is covered in two chapters. The next covers the surgical management of infected joints and arthroplasties. This chapter covers the surgical techniques designed to address the problems encountered when managing osteomyelitis: necrotic tissue; soft tissue defects; dead space; and loss of bony continuity. In most cases a specific technique addresses more than one problem (eg, tissue transfer eliminates dead space and soft tissue defects). The techniques are broadly organized into six groups: débridement; manipulation, or transfer, of vascularized tissue; antibiotic spacers and antibiotic pumps; autogenous cancellous bone grafting; external fixation with static or dynamic frames; and internal fixation with plates or nails.

Débridement

Débridement of necrotic tissue and foreign material is the starting point in the management of bone and joint infections. Necrotic bone and foreign material provide surfaces to which bacteria adhere, increasing their resistance to antibiotics, humoral factors (e.g., antibodies

and complement), and white blood cells. This has two clinical implications. (1) It may be very difficult to control the progression of an infection complicated by the presence of necrotic tissue and foreign bodies. Cellulitis, osteolysis, purulent drainage, and pain may result in permanent loss of function and necessitate complex reconstructive procedures. (2) Adherent bacteria may remain dormant, and there may be no clinical signs of infection, until a stimulus activates the bacteria. The bacteria begin to replicate, and infection becomes clinically evident. Therefore, in cases in which infection is progressing uncontrollably, or in which cure or permanent suppression of infection is the goal, all necrotic soft tissue, bone, and foreign material must be surgically débrided. Carrying the principle of surgical débridement to the extreme leads to the removal of viable tissue and implants which are vital to the function of a limb or are providing necessary stability. This results in loss of function, or even amputation. The central problem is to identify tissue which is necrotic, and implants which are not serving a constructive purpose.

Saucerization or externalization of infected wounds is an extension of surgical débridement. The concept is that by leaving débrided wounds open widely, through excision of overhanging soft tissue and bone, the wound drains freely, abscesses do not form, and cellulitis slowly resolves. Saucerization is the classic method of management of bone and joint infections and was in use long before the advent of antibiotics. Today, the use of saucerization is limited to areas in which it will result in an acceptable loss of function, such as the diaphysis of the tibia or femur. Saucerization of periarticular infections is performed only as a last resort because it results in ankylosis of the joint. Infections involving the proximal femur and hip are usually not suitable for this technique, because the excision of overlying soft tissue necessary to open the wound widely results in unacceptable loss of function. Saucerization in a less radical form (i.e., packing a wound open) is useful as a salvage procedure, to temporize and delay definitive wound management, or when we find that débridement has resulted in a greater defect than anticipated. The initial step of a Papineau procedure can be considered externalization of an infected wound.[1]

A number of reported series, most from before 1975, illustrate the effectiveness of this conceptually simple technique. Most notably, Knight and Wood reported 23 cases in which osteomyelitis with the infected bone in continuity was managed with débridement and saucerization followed by split thickness skin grafting.[2] Several defects were later reconstructed by excising the skin graft and filling the cavity with autogenous cancellous graft. The overall good results, 19 patients with long term suppression of infection, and the astonishing case reports documented in this paper underline the effectiveness of radical débridement and saucerization. Kelly et al, and more recently Evans and Davies, and Gupta reported similar results using the same technique.[3–5]

Technique: débridement

Necrotic soft tissue is easily recognized. It does not bleed when cut, and differs in appearance from surrounding viable tissue. Necrotic muscle will not contract when stimulated by electrocautery or pinching with a forceps. Hematoma is considered to be necrotic and is removed by irrigation and curettage. The viability of tendons and ligaments is difficult to assess, and unnecessary débridement is associated with significant loss of function. This problem is most frequently encountered with infections involving the patellar ligament, and Achilles tendon. One way to approach this problem is with staged procedures. At the first operation, all fragmented tissue is removed. Tendon or ligament which appears structurally intact is left undisturbed. The wound is kept moist with wet dressings, which are changed daily. Further fragmentation of tendon or ligament necessitates a second débridement. If the tendon or ligament remains intact, and granulation tissue forms on its surface, it is viable, and is covered with a free or local soft tissue transfer. Sinus tracts consist of viable tissue, but harbor large numbers of bacteria. They are excised if excision will not result in a more difficult reconstructive procedure. When they are left in situ, they involute spontaneously as the infection is brought under control.

The surgical exposure for débridement of necrotic bone is tailored to each case. The approach must be extensive enough to expose all suspect areas and yet it must be designed to minimize devitalization of tissue which has been compromised by previous surgery. Usually it is best to use previous incisions when débriding posttraumatic or postsurgical infections, and approaches with which the surgeon is familiar when débriding hematogenous infections. During the surgical exposure and débridement care is taken to minimize further devitalization of bone.

The vascular supply of diaphyseal bone is via periosteal vessels and nutrient arteries in the medullary canal. The metaphysis is supplied by metaphyseal vessels which perforate the cortex of the metaphysis. It is important to minimize damage to these sources of vascularity. Therefore, the technique of "subperiosteal exposure" is seldom utilized. Retractors which result in soft tissue stripping (eg, Hohman, Bennet, and Criego retractors) are avoided, as they may damage the periosteum, or strip it from the underlying bone. Sequential reaming of a medullary canal destroys the medullary vessels, and is therefore avoided in most cases. The one instance in which we routinely use reaming is following removal of an infected intramedullary nail. The alternative is to unroof the medullary canal in order to débride it adequately. This is reserved for cases in which there is persistent infection following nail removal and reaming. In these cases, the surgical procedure can usually be limited to one portion of the bone (eg, proximal middle or distal third of the tibia) and is not as extensive as it would be if done as a primary procedure. The combination of periosteal stripping and reaming of the medullary canal must be avoided, as it will result in segmental devitalization of the cortex.

Viable bone is identified by active "pin point" bleeding from osteons. Bleeding can only be seen if a tourniquet is not being used. High speed burrs or osteotomes are used to remove necrotic bone. The use of high speed burrs minimizes the risk of fracture; however, the burr will cause thermal necrosis if not constantly irrigated. The use of osteotomes increases the chance of fracturing a bone already attenuated by débridement, but there is no risk of thermal necrosis. The bone is irrigated throughout the débridement to clear its surface of blood and debris so that the pin point bleeders can be identified. It may be difficult to determine whether dysvascular bone and scar should be removed. We tend to err on the side of débridement at the cost of requiring more extensive secondary procedures for closure and management of dead space. As with soft tissue débridement, the presence of granulation four to seven days after the initial débridement indicates a healthy vascularized wound.

Foreign bodies serve as a surface to which bacteria adhere. Indications for leaving an implant in an infected area are: when tne implant is providing stability of a fracture or nonunion; when removal of the implant will require such an extensive surgical exposure or removal of bone that less harm is done by leaving it in place (eg, a broken screw in the femoral head); and infected arthroplasties in which extremely high concentrations of antibiotic can be achieved within the joint capsule. When an implant fails to provide stability it is removed. Radiographic signs of loss of stability are: broken screws, plates, or nails; the "windshield wiper" sign; and a change in alignment seen on stress radiographs. Broken intramedullary nails are removed by closed technique if possible, ie, the nonunion is not opened. I have found the following technique to be successful in the majority of cases.

Through the original incision, the extractor is attached to the proximal fragment of the nail. The proximal fragment is removed. A beaded guide wire is inserted down the medullary canal, through the nail, and out of the tip (Fig. 6.1a). In cases in which the nail has been in place for a year or more this can be difficult owing to tissue ingrowth within the nail. The proximal canal is reamed 1 mm larger than the diameter of the nail (Fig. 6.1b). This prevents the edges of the remaining fragment of the nail from catching on the sides of the medullary canal during extraction. A smooth guide wire is inserted down the nail and out of the tip, "stacking" the nail (Fig. 6.1c). The bead tipped guide wire is now extracted along with the nail (Fig. 6.1d). This technique cannot be used with solid core nails, or when deformity of the bone will prevent removal of the nail. In these cases, the nonunion site is "taken down". The distal fragment of the nail is extracted through the nonunion site.

Follow up: débridement

Débridement is combined with other procedures, eg: primary closure; saucerization (see below); external fixation; or tissue transfer. The follow up care of the débrided infected wound always involves dressing changes to confirm that an abscess has not formed, but otherwise is

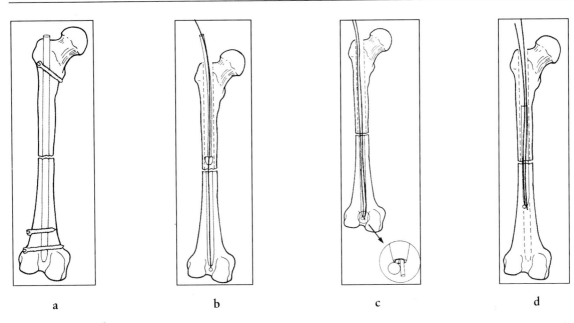

a   b   c   d

Figure 6.1 (a–d)

Removal of a broken nail. See text for explanation.

dependent upon which procedures were performed in conjunction with the débridement.

Technique: saucerization

When it is elected to manage an infected wound by saucerization, it is critical that an adequate débridement be performed. All overlying bone and soft tissue is excised; this may result in a segmental defect of the bone which requires stabilization with an external fixator. Casting and then windowing the cast to obtain exposure of the wound is not recommended, as the cast quickly becomes soiled with wound drainage. The wound is packed loosely with gauze soaked in a topical antibiotic.

Follow up: saucerization

Dressing changes start no later than the second postoperative day, and are then performed daily.

The type of dressing is based on the surgeon's preference. Reconstruction of the defect is undertaken when the wound has started to granulate, and ranges in complexity from something as simple as split thickness skin grafting or filling the defect with autogenous cancellous bone (Papineau procedure), to distraction osteogenesis or free tissue transfer.

Complications: débridement

The complications of débridement are: inadequate débridement, resulting in persistent infection; and excessive débridement, resulting in instability or significant loss of function. Inadequate débridement is most frequently inadvertent. A small area of necrotic bone or a foreign body is left behind because it is not identified. The best way to avoid this is simply to be careful. The remedy is a second operative procedure to redébride the area. Occasionally, an inadequate débridement is performed because, in the surgeon's judgment, the loss of function which would result from a thorough débridement is less desirable than persistent infection.

Manipulation of vascularized soft tissue

Soft tissue is manipulated to increase local vascularity, fill dead space created by the débridement, and to close the wound. The relative vascularity of local tissue is important. The débrided wound is often hypovascular, and soft tissue flaps which are parasitic (eg, cross leg flaps, or split thickness skin grafts) or which have precarious intrinsic circulation (eg, fasciocutaneous flaps) are associated with a high incidence of failure. When using transferred tissue to fill dead space it is critical that no dead space is left under the transfer. It may be necessary to contour the bed or the tissue to be transferred in order to create a better fit. The three types of closure which are most useful in the management of bone and joint infections are: primary closure; local muscle transfer; and free soft tissue transfer.

Primary closure

Primary closure denotes approximating the wound edges with sutures. Primary closure of an infected wound runs counter to historical surgical principles. The risk of closure is that an infected cavity is created, and develops into an abscess. Today, administration of antibiotics specifically directed at the pathogenic organisms, management of dead space with spacers or autogenous bone graft, and adequate transcutaneous suction drainage, make primary closure of selected infected wounds an excellent method of coverage. Primary closure is performed only when the infection is under control, and only when it can be accomplished with minimal tension on the surrounding soft tissue.

Technique: primary closure

Dead space must be occupied with beads or bone graft prior to closure. Large bore suction drains are left in all wounds, unless the wound is so superficial that adequate drainage will occur through the suture line. As a general rule buried sutures are not used. Exceptions to this rule are: when not using buried sutures results in dead space between the sides of the wound; when not approximating deep tissues results in tension on the skin edges; and when not approximating deep tissues results in disability or loss of function (eg, the medial retinaculum must be closed after draining an infected total knee, or the patella will dislocate laterally). Vertical mattress sutures are used to close the skin because they minimize the amount of subcutaneous dead space. Monofilament proline, nylon or wire are used, as they cause minimal inflammation.

Follow up: primary closure

The patient is followed very carefully in the perioperative period for signs of an abscess. These signs are: swelling; pain; temperature spikes; and cellulitis. If there is any doubt, skin sutures are removed over the most suspicious area and the wound is probed. In cases in which buried sutures have been utilized the wound must be explored in the operating room. If an abscess has accumulated, all sutures are removed, and the wound is débrided and packed open.

If all goes well and there are no signs of an abscess, the drains are removed after drainage has decreased to less than 30 ml per day. If drainage does not decrease to this level the drains are left in place for three to four weeks. This allows enough time for the incision to heal and a sinus tract to develop around the drainage tubes. This minimizes the chance of drainage occurring through the surgical incision, and the scar becoming inverted and macerated. Antibiotics are continued for a minimum of three weeks following primary closure, to protect the skin and soft tissue.

Local muscle transfer

Ger was one of the first to advocate muscle transfer to cover the exposed infected tibia.[6,7] In 1970 he and Efron reported nine patients with chronic osteomyelitis of the tibia managed with débridement and gastrocnemius or soleus muscle transposition. It appears that the bone was in continuity in all cases. Suppression of infection was achieved in eight patients. Ger and Efron attributed this high rate of success to the muscle transfer, which "allows radical removal of diseased tissue, obliterates the dead space, improves the blood supply and allows satisfactory skin cover".

Other authors have extrapolated from this work and described other muscles which can be transposed to cover defects in other areas. Stern and Carey reported a series of 19 patients who underwent local transfer of the latissimus dorsi to the shoulder.[8] The latissimus dorsi was detached from its insertion and origin and rotated on its neurovascular pedicle. The majority of procedures were performed in order to increase elbow flexion (i.e., elbow flexorplasty). However, among the 19 patients were six with chronic osteomyelitis or septic arthritis, in whom the transfer was performed to achieve soft tissue coverage following débridement. There were no failures in this group. The vastus lateralis has been transferred on its vascular pedicle to cover defects around the hip.[9] Collins et al reported seven patients with infected hip implants who were managed with débridement and rotation of the vastus lateralis into the defect.[10] The infection was successfully suppressed in all cases. Little et al described rotation of the gluteus medius and tensor fascia lata to cover defects about the hip.[11]

The principle of local muscle transfer is to dissect free a muscle, or portion of a muscle, from surrounding tissue, while preserving its vascular pedicle. The end result is a muscle which can be used to cover a neighboring defect. The advantage of local muscle transfer is that, unlike free soft tissue transfer, the procedure is simple, and does not require any special expertise or equipment. The disadvantages of local muscle transfer is that the number and types of transfers are limited, and therefore not all areas can be adequately covered. The distal tibia is an example. Successful local muscle transfer requires a knowledge of the vascular supply of the muscle to be transferred, and an understanding of which transfer should be used in a given situation.

Technique: gastrocnemius muscle transfer

Either the medial or lateral half of the gastrocnemius muscles can be transferred. The medial gastrocnemius muscle is the most useful for local tissue transfers and can be rotated to cover defects extending from the patella to the junction of the proximal and middle thirds of the tibia. The vascular supply of the medial gastrocnemius is from the sural artery, and enters the under surface (anatomically, the anterior surface) of the muscle in the popliteal fossae. The lateral gastrocnemius muscle transfer is used primarily to cover defects over the lateral aspect of the knee. The usefulness of this flap is limited by the length of the lateral head of the gastrocnemius, and by the presence of the fibula. Both of these factors limit the arc of rotation of the flap. The vascular supply of the lateral head is similar to that of the medial head, and enters the muscle in the popliteal fossae.

For a medial gastrocnemius muscle transfer, the patient is supine with the leg and foot prepped and draped free. A tourniquet is used. The skin incision is parallel and 1 cm posterior to the posterior medial border of the tibia. It extends from the level of the distal pole of the patella to the junction of the distal and middle third of the tibia. The gastrocnemius is easily freed from the overlying subcutaneous tissue

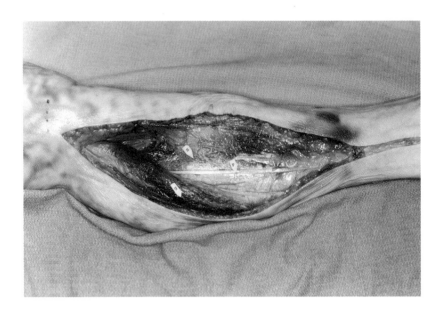

Figure 6.2

Transfer of the gastrocnemius muscle. The interval between the soleus muscle, "S", and the gastrocnemius, "g", is confirmed by the presence of the plantaris tendon, "P".

with blunt dissection. The interval between the soleus and the gastrocnemius is identified and these two muscles are separated in the proximal third of the calf. The tendon of the plantaris muscle is found between the gastrocnemius and soleus and confirms that the correct interval has been entered (Fig. 6.2). The raphe of the gastrocnemius is identified approximately in the sagittal midline of the muscle. It is easier to identify the raphe proximally, where the medial and lateral heads merge, than distally near their insertion on the Achilles tendon. The raphe is gently separated with scissors and blunt dissection, from proximally to distally. At the musculotendinous junction, the medial half of the Achilles tendon is divided. A suture is passed through the distal tip of the flap and is used for retraction. The dissection of the raphe is now carried proximally as needed to increase the arc of rotation. As the dissection proceeds proximally, adequate exposure is mandatory to visualize and protect the sural artery (Fig. 6.3). The dissection can be carried to the origin of the medial gastrocnemius from the medial femoral condyle. The tourniquet is deflated and hemostasis is achieved. The flap is rotated to cover the defect (Fig. 6.4). If more

coverage is needed, the fascia on the under surface of the muscle can be incised in line with its fibers at 1 cm intervals to increase the width of the transfer. Horizontal mattress sutures are used to hold the gastrocnemius in the desired location. A split thickness skin graft is applied, and the skin incision is closed over a drain. A bulky dressing is applied to the extremity.

The technique of lateral gastrocnemius transfer is similar to that of the medial gastrocnemius transfer. The patient is positioned supine with a large bolster under the ipsilateral hip, or on his or her side, with the operated side up. The skin incision is parallel and 1 cm posterior to the fibula. The posterior surface of the gastrocnemius is freed from the overlying subcutaneous tissue. The peroneal nerve is identified and protected as it passes around the neck of the fibula. The interval between the soleus and the gastrocnemius is identified (Fig. 6.5). The gastrocnemius is split along its raphe, and the lateral half of the Achilles tendon is divided at its musculotendinous junction. The raphe can be dissected further proximally as needed. Closure is identical to that following a medial gastrocnemius transfer.

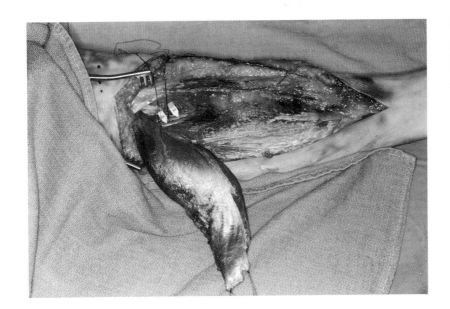

Figure 6.3

Proximal dissection is performed carefully to avoid injury to the sural artery, "sa", and tibial nerve, "tn".

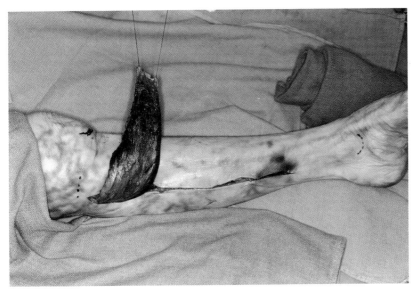

Figure 6.4

The medial head of the gastrocnemius is rotated to cover the defect.

Follow up: gastrocnemius muscle transfer

The drain is removed and the dressing is changed according to the surgeon's preference. In the immediate postoperative period, the patient must be carefully examined daily for signs and symptoms of an abscess developing beneath the flap. The leg is kept elevated two to four weeks after surgery. At two to four weeks, active range of motion of the ankle and knee is begun. The mattress sutures holding the flap in place are left in for a minimum of four weeks, to prevent delayed retraction of the flap.

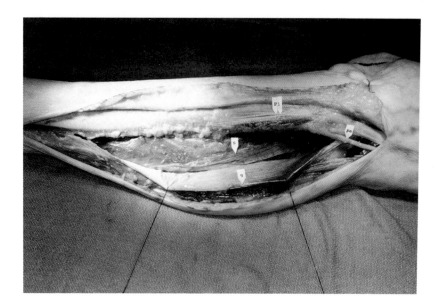

Figure 6.5

Transfer of the lateral head of the gastrocnemius, "g". The interval between the soleus, "S", and gastrocnemius is identified. The peroneal nerve, "pn", is protected as it passes distal to the neck of the fibula. The peroneus longus, "Pl", is seen anteriorly.

Technique: soleus muscle transfer

The soleus muscle transfer is the most useful local tissue transfer for defects of the middle third of the tibia. Its usefulness is somewhat limited by the pattern of its vascular supply, which is segmental in the proximal third of the muscle and primarily from the posterior tibial artery. In addition, because the soleus blends gradually with the Achilles tendon, as opposed to the medial head of the gastrocnemius, which has a more discreet insertion, the dissection of the muscle distally from the tendon is difficult. The soleus can be transferred medially or laterally; however, the medial transfer is more useful, as the lateral transfer is hindered by the fibula. Indications for lateral transfer include: patients with a lateral tibial defect; a mid-third tibial defect with destruction of the medial side of the soleus; and patients in whom the fibula has been resected.

For a medial soleus muscle transfer, the patient is positioned as described for a medial gastrocnemius transfer. The skin incision extends from below the level of the knee joint to the ankle and is 1 cm posterior to the posterior medial border of the tibia. The plane between the soleus and gastrocnemius is identified and opened. The plantaris tendon is found in this intermuscular interval. Anteriorly, the interval between the soleus and the muscles of the deep posterior compartment is identified, and confirmed by the presence of the posterior tibial artery and nerve (Fig. 6.6). The soleus is dissected off the Achilles tendon. Sutures are placed in the distal end of the muscle and are used for retraction of the muscle. The dissection is carried as far proximally as needed. As the dissection proceeds proximally, vascular pedicles, or perforators, to the muscle from the posterior tibial artery are identified. One, or at most two, of these pedicles can be ligated to increase the arc of rotation of the soleus (Fig. 6.7). Suture ligation, as opposed to electrocautery, is necessary because of the proximity of the posterior tibial artery. If only the medial half of the soleus is required, the muscle is split in line with its fibers, and the lateral half is left in situ. The muscle is rotated to the desired position and the wounds are closed as described for the medial gastrocnemius transfer (Fig. 6.8).

For a lateral soleus transfer, the patient is positioned on his or her side with the entire leg and foot scrubbed and draped free. The skin incision

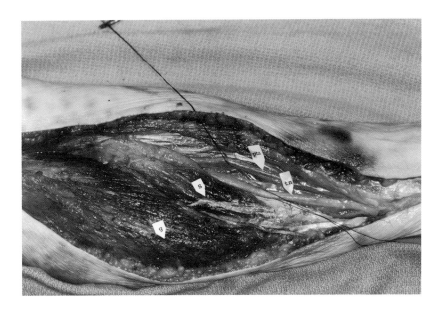

Figure 6.6

Transfer of the medial heal of the soleus. The anterior surface of the soleus, "S", is confirmed by the presence of the posterior artery, "pta", and tibial nerve, "tn". The gastrocnemius, g, can also be seen.

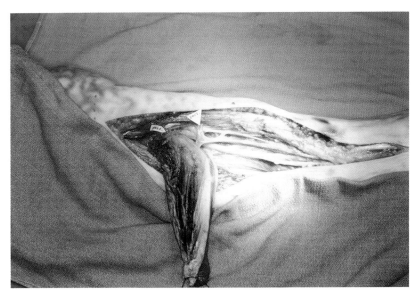

Figure 6.7

As the dissection of the medial head of the soleus proceeds proximally, perforators from the posterior tibial artery "perf", are encountered. One, or at most two, of these can be ligated.

is just posterior to the fibula and extends from below the level of the knee to the ankle joint. The soleus is located between the peroneus longus and the gastrocnemius. The interval between the gastrocnemius and soleus is opened and the soleus is dissected off the Achilles tendon distally. The muscle is freed from distally to proximally; this is difficult because the fibula obstructs the view of the medial side of the muscle (Fig. 6.9). Care is taken to protect the posterior tibial

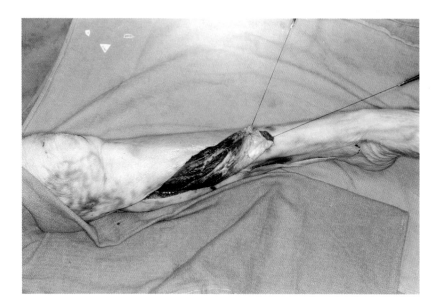

Figure 6.8

The medial head of the soleus is rotated to cover defects of the mid-third of the tibia.

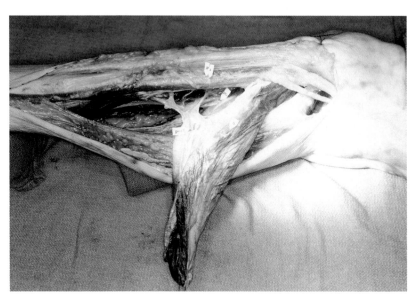

Figure 6.9

Transfer of the lateral head of the soleus. The muscle is rotated on the perforators "perf", which originate from the posterior tibial artery, "pta". The peroneus longus, "Pl", is directly anterior to the soleus "S".

artery. The soleus is freed proximally enough to cover the defect. The tourniquet is released and bleeders identified and ligated. The muscle is transferred to its desired location and held in place with mattress sutures.

Follow up: soleus muscle transfer

In the perioperative period, the patient is carefully observed for signs of an expanding hematoma. If this occurs the wound must be explored and hemostasis obtained. The remainder of the

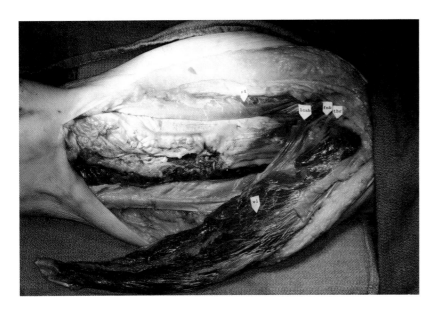

Figure 6.10

Transfer of the vastus lateralis (vl). The muscle has been detached distally and elevated from the vastus intermedius and rectus femoris (rf) up to its arterial supply, a branch of the lateral circumflex artery, "lcab", and its nerve supply branches of the femoral nerve, "fnb and tbr".

follow up care is identical to that described for gastrocnemius transfer.

Technique: vastus lateralis transfer

The vastus lateralis transfer is useful in covering defects around the hip. It is used most frequently to manage persistent infection following resection of an infected arthroplasty. The vascular supply of the vastus lateralis is primarily from a descending branch of the lateral circumflex femoral artery. It enters the vastus lateralis at the junction of its proximal and middle thirds. There may be ancillary vessels originating from the perforators which enter the vastus lateralis in its distal third, making it impossible to transfer this portion of the muscle proximally.

The patient is in the lateral decubitus position. The hip and leg are draped free. The skin incision parallels and is posterior to the lateral border of the rectus femoris. It starts over the greater trochanter, and extends distally, curving anteriorly to a point 6 cm proximal to the patella. The fascia lata is opened in line with the incision. The vastus lateralis is freed from the fascia lata and the lateral intermuscular septum with blunt dissection. The interval between the rectus and lateralis is identified and opened distally. The tendinous insertion of the lateralis is incised 8 cm proximal to the patella. The lateralis is elevated from distally to proximally off the femur and vastus intermedius. The artery to the vastus lateralis is encountered approximately two thirds of the way up the muscle (8–10 cm distal to the anterior superior iliac spine), where it runs between the vastus intermedius and rectus femoris. The vessels are mobilized with careful blunt and sharp dissection to increase the arc of rotation (Fig. 6.10). A significant portion of the distal vastus lateralis may receive its vascular supply from perforating arteries. When this occurs the fibers of the vastus lateralis are found to blend with the fibers of the vastus intermedius. Using sharp dissection, these fibers should be separated from the remainder of the vastus lateralis and left with the vastus intermedius. The muscle can be turned 180° on itself in order to fill a defect at the hip (Fig. 6.11). The muscle is securely sutured in place and a suction drain is left beneath it.

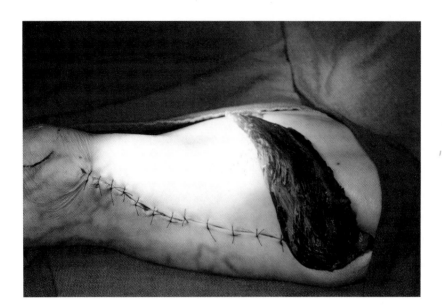

Figure 6.11

The vastus lateralis can now be rotated to fill proximal defects.

Follow up: vastus lateralis transfer

The patient has bedrest for two to three weeks, after which weight bearing is allowed. The sutures are left in place at least four weeks. The drains are left in until drainage is less than 30 ml per day.

Free tissue transfer

Free tissue transfer has the theoretical advantage that a well vascularized soft tissue envelope is more able to clear a bacterial inoculum successfully than a hypovascular envelope. This technique is of particular value when there is no tissue available for local transfer, either because of the location of the defect (eg, the distal tibia) or because tissue which could be transferred has been traumatized. The most frequently transferred soft tissues are the latissimus dorsi, the rectus abdominis and the gracilis. The initial reports by May and Savage, and Mathes et al, describing the use of free tissue transfer in

the management of osteomyelitis were overly optimistic, claiming close to a 100% cure rate.[12,13] As more experience was gained, the initial enthusiasm was tempered with reality. Weiland et al reported a series of 33 patients with osteomyelitis managed with free tissue transfer.[14] Of these 33 patients, 23 had a segmental defect of the bone. In six of these the tissue transfer failed, and nine patients developed recurrent sepsis. This report emphasizes the high incidence of complications and failures of free tissue transfer in the management of infected segmental defects. Gordon and Chui reported the results of free tissue transfer followed by delayed bone grafting, if necessary, in 14 patients.[15] The authors felt that the soft tissue transfer resulted in suppression of the infection, allowing successful management of "the underlying osseous defect". They found that the six patients without a segmental defect all healed their nonunions without bone grafting. The remaining eight patients had a defect of the tibia at least 3 cm in length. The defect was managed with a tibiofibular synostosis, autogenous grafting or free fibular transfer. Two of the most severely involved patients eventually underwent below knee amputation; the remaining six healed. The authors' concept of handling infected segmental defects in a staged manner (stage I, control of infection with a free flap; stage II, reconstruction of osseous defect) is unique and no doubt accounts for their excellent results. The technique of free tissue transfer will not be described.

Complications: soft tissue manipulation

The most significant complication of soft tissue manipulation is necrosis of the soft tissue. Foremost among the factors leading to necrosis of the soft tissue are excessive tension and uncontrolled infection. The best way to avoid excessive tension is experience. Usually, by the time excessive tension has been identified as the cause of tissue necrosis, revision or suture removal is not successful in salvaging the tissue transferred. An uncontrolled infection will threaten transferred soft tissue. To decrease the incidence of uncontrolled infection the soft tissue transfer is performed only after adequate débridement has been achieved and the wound has stabilized. An integral part of the procedure is to provide adequate drainage of the area beneath the transferred tissue, to prevent formation of an abscess. If adequate drainage has not been achieved, eg, a drain has inadvertently been discontinued, the wound is débrided and a drain reinserted. In cases in which there is worsening cellulitis, cultures are rechecked. Occasionally a "second look" procedure is necessary to rule out residual necrotic bone or tissue.

Manipulation of vascularized bone

Vascularized bone transfer differs from reconstruction with autogenous cancellous grafts or allografts in that the segment of transferred tissue is living. Theoretically, living bone is more resistant to infection and will heal more quickly to the bone ends. In reality, healing of the graft to the bone ends is not reliable and frequently supplemental autogenous cancellous grafting is required.

There are two techniques of vascularized bone transfer: the Huntington fibular transfer; and free vascularized bone transfer. In 1905 Huntington described centralization of the fibula and fixation of it to the tibia, in effect local transfer of the fibula.[16] Disadvantages of the Huntington procedure are that: prolonged immobilization and nonweight bearing are necessary to protect the synostosis; the number of candidates for this procedure is limited by the fact that an intact fibula is required; hypertrophy of the fibula is necessary to achieve a good functional result; and segmental tibial defects with a very short proximal or distal segment are difficult to manage with this method. An extensive experience with the technique of local transfer of the fibula has not been reported. The two largest series reviewed a total of 12 cases.[17,18] Posterolateral bone grafting can be thought of as a modification of the Huntington fibular transfer. In this technique bone graft is placed between the tibia and fibula, producing a synostosis. However, the fibula is not centralized, and we have found that the eccentrically loaded fibula is not strong enough to withstand weight bearing in cases in which there is a segmental tibial defect. For this reason we do not use posterolateral bone grafting for segmental defects, and reserve this technique for patients with simple nonunions.

The second technique of vascularized bone transfer is free vascularized bone transfer.[19–22] This technique involves the mobilization of a segment of bone with its vascular pedicle. The vascular pedicle is anastomosed to nearby arteries and veins at the site of the defect. A defect of 6 cm is the minimum indication. The disadvantages of free vascularized bone grafts include: donor site morbidity; the extensive and technically difficult surgical procedure; and the protracted period of nonweight bearing necessary to protect the synostosis sites.

Han et al reviewed their results of 160 vascularized bone transfers in the management of skeletal defects.[23] Of note is that although none of these patients had an active infection at the time of tissue transfer, the single worst prognostic factor was a history of infection. Of the 60 patients with a history of infection, only 27 healed after the first procedure. An additional 19 patients healed after secondary procedures. Ten of the 60 patients eventually underwent amputation. Based on the number of secondary procedures required, better results were obtained with a free fibula (17% required secondary procedures) than a free iliac crest transfer (32% required secondary procedures). The authors conclude that free tissue transfer which includes a segment of vascularized bone is a viable alternative in the reconstruction of infected segmental defects because "reliable reconstructive techniques are lacking and amputation is often the only alternative". Whether transfer of fibula or iliac crest is more effective is not entirely clear.

Salibian et al reported the results of vascularized iliac crest transfer in the management of segmental defects of the upper and lower extremity. Nine patients had actively infected defects.[24] An external fixator was used to stabilize the extremity postoperatively. There were no outright failures, although the authors modified their technique and recommended osteomuscular transfers instead of osteomusculocutaneous transfers. Unlike Han et al's series, infection did not adversely affect the prognosis. They conclude that iliac crest transfer is indicated for defects less than 9 cm in length, and that larger defects should be managed with a free fibula.

Vascularized bone transfer is used to manage defects of bones other than the tibia. Weiland and Daniel reported eight patients, six of whom underwent a free fibula transfer, and two a free iliac crest transfer for defects of the radius femur and tibia.[21] Jupiter et al reported four infected femoral defects managed with free vascularized fibular transfer.[25] All four patients healed their

nonunions and had no further signs of infection.

Four principles of vascularized bone transfer emerge from these series. First, segmental defects of the tibia are more difficult to manage than segmental defects of other bones. Second, a staged procedure yields the best results. The initial stage is suppression of infection with bony stabilization, soft tissue reconstruction, and antibiotic administration. The second stage is bony reconstruction. Third, the most important determinant of which transfer, fibula or iliac crest, has the greatest chance of success, is the familiarity of the surgeon with the technique. However, active infection is a relative indication for iliac crest transfer instead of fibular transfer. Fourth, vascularized bone transfer is an effective method of managing segmental defects in general; the transferred bone can be expected to undergo hypertrophy to the extent that it can bear physiologic loads without fracturing, regardless of where it is implanted.

Technique: Huntington fibular transfer

A virgin area of the tibia proximal to the segmental defect is chosen, and through an anterior incision a notch is made in the lateral cortex of the tibia. Similarly, the distal tibia is notched for acceptance of the fibular graft. Posterolateral incisions are used to expose the fibula at the level of the synostosis. A transverse osteotomy of the proximal fibula is completed just proximal to the notch in the tibia. The transverse osteotomy of the distal fibula is made at a level just distal to the distal tibial notch. Using both incisions, the fibula is wedged into the recipient notch sites, and locked into place. The fibula is fixed to the tibia with screws and the synostosis is reinforced with cancellous grafts.

Alternatively, the procedure can be performed in two stages, as originally described by Huntington. The proximal tibiofibular synostosis comprises the first stage. Following union at the proximal synostosis site, the distal synostosis is performed.

Follow up: Huntington fibular transfer

A nonweight bearing long leg cast is applied until the synostosis sites are united, usually three to four months following a one stage procedure. If the procedure was performed in two stages, a second immobilization period of, three to four months, is necessary. Once union has occurred both proximally and distally, partial weight bearing in a short leg walking cast is maintained for approximately two to three months while the fibula hypertrophies. At five to seven months after a one stage Huntington fibular transfer, weight bearing is gradually advanced to full.

The technique of free vascularized fibula and iliac crest transfer will not be described.

Complications: free vascularized bone transfer

The complications of free vascularized bone transfer are failure of union between the transferred bone and the recipient bone, and fracture of the transferred bone. A flare up of infection can also threaten the transferred tissue, and is managed as described above, under "Complications: soft tissue manipulation". Failure of union between the transferred bone and recipient bone is managed by immobilization and bone grafting with autogenous cancellous bone. When necessary, internal fixation in the form of plates, screws and wires is revised, or an external fixator is applied. Fracture of the transferred bone is managed with casting or external fixation. Intramedullary nails are not feasible, and plates will serve as an additional stress riser. In my experience most fractures of the transferred bone are low energy, minimally displaced and frequently heal with noninvasive management.

Antibiotic spacers and pumps

Antibiotic spacers and pumps deliver local antibiotics directly to the infected area. Antibiotic spacers deliver a limited amount of drug, and can only be used when there is a significant volume of dead space. Pumps deliver an unlimited amount of drug, and can be used even when there is no dead space, but they are not an effective method of dead space management. The concept of dead space is an important one. It is defined as the space left in a wound after closure. In the surgery of bone and joint infections, dead space is frequently created by the débridement of necrotic tissue and the removal of implants. This space quickly fills with exudate and hematoma in the postoperative period. If bacteria are present, the exudate and hematoma provide nutrients and an environment ideal for replication. The problem is compounded by the fact that penetration of this large hematoma–seroma by antibiotics and humoral elements (eg, antibodies and complement) and cellular elements (eg, polymorphonuclear leukocytes) of the immune system is limited. For these reasons, dead space must be minimized. Methods of dead space management are: not closing the wound, in essence saucerizing, or externalizing, the defect; modifying wound closure to fill the dead space (eg, closure with a free tissue transfer); or occupying the space with something (ie, bone graft, beads, or an absorbable spacer) that prevents the accumulation of hematoma.

The PMMA–antibiotic beads serve three purposes. They fill dead space, preventing it being filled with serum and blood. They maintain dead space, making it easier to bone graft or perform a revision arthroplasty, and they deliver antibiotics to the surrounding cavity. It is key to remember that PMMA–antibiotic beads are a method of temporary dead space management. In most cases they must be removed and the dead space occupied with a tissue transfer, or a bone graft. A PMMA–antibiotic spacer is frequently used when infected total knee arthroplasties are managed with two stage revision; this is covered in Chapter 7.

Technique: PMMA–antibiotic spacer

PMMA–antibiotic spacers are in the form of beads or larger blocks. The fabrication of antibiotic methylmethacrylate beads and their use as an antibiotic delivery system is covered in Chapter 5. The beads are packed into the débrided wound. Wound closure is mandatory to minimize the emergence of bacterial strains which are resistant to the antibiotics used in the beads.

Follow up: PMMA–antibiotic spacers

Systemic antibiotics are initiated during the implantation of the beads or block and continued a minimum of three weeks. Administration of antibiotics during implantation of the beads is necessary because the beads do not occupy all the dead space. Theoretically, we would like antibiotics to be in the hematoma surrounding the beads. Continued administration of antibiotics systemically is necessary because the local levels of antibiotic due to elution of antibiotic from the beads decreases very quickly following implantation of the beads.

Beads are usually removed between three and six weeks after they have been implanted. If the beads are left in place longer than six weeks, they may become entrapped in scar tissue, and their removal will require considerable dissection. To remove the beads, part of the incision is opened, the strand of beads is found and, as atraumatically as possible, gently teased from the wound. The sides of the cavity are curetted of organized hematoma and, if indicated, specimens are sent for culture. The walls of the cavity are carefully inspected for necrotic bone that may have been missed in prior débridements. Reconstruction of the defect can now proceed with a soft tissue

transfer, or more frequently bone grafting, as described in the next section.

Antibiotic pumps

With local antibiotic administration via an implantable pump, extremely high concentrations of antibiotic are obtained at the site of infection. At the same time the systemic concentration of antibiotic is well below the level at which toxicity occurs. Local antibiotic delivery via an implanted pump can be used in conjunction with PMMA–antibiotic beads, intramedullary nails, and external fixation.

Technique: pump implantation

Amikacin, tobramycin, clindamycin, and aztreonam are the only antibiotics which are stable in the pump. Vancomycin and the cephalosporins are not stable and cannot be used in the pump.[26] Amikacin in a concentration of 50 mg/ml is the drug used most frequently in the pump. The pump is implanted in the lower quadrant of the abdomen, usually the ipsilateral lower quadrant in cases in which the infection is distal to the knee, and the contralateral lower quadrant when the femur or hip is infected. When scrubbing and draping the patient, care is taken to avoid contaminating the pump site with material from the infected area. Two separate surgical scrubs are performed, and the infected area draped out of the sterile field. First, the pump is implanted through a transverse incision at the level of the umbilicus. A pocket is formed superficial to the preabdominal fascia. Meticulous hemostasis is maintained to prevent a postoperative hematoma, which could become infected. The outflow catheters are pulled distally through the subcutaneous tissue with a tendon passer; they are brought through the skin, coiled and held in place with an adhesive drape. The pump site is closed and covered with an impermeable drape prior to surgical manipulation of the infected area. Following the surgical procedure of the infected area, the outflow catheters are pulled through the subcutaneous tissue and inserted into the infected area. Positioning of the catheters is empiric and should give the best spread of antibiotic. The catheter tips can be sewn into place with fine absorbable suture, to prevent their migration. The infected wound is closed over a drain. Leaving the wound open increases the chance of superinfection with resistant organisms.

Follow-up: antibiotic pump

Systemic antibiotics are administered in the perioperative period to minimize the chance of pump site infection and to treat the cellulitis which is so frequently associated with bone and joint infections. The drain is left in place until its output is less than 10 ml per 8 hours. The antibiotic level of the drainage is determined to confirm that the pump is delivering antibiotics to the infected area. The pump is filled as an outpatient procedure at weekly intervals. The timing of pump removal is based on the clinical course.

Complications: antibiotic spacers and pumps

The complications of spacers are difficulty in removing them and wound dehiscence. Beads are less difficult to remove within six weeks of implantation. After six weeks they are entrapped in scar. When wound dehiscence occurs the beads should be removed, to prevent infection with resistant organisms.

The complications of antibiotic pumps are: migration of the catheters from the infected area; the pump "flips", making refill impossible; infection of the pump or catheters; and superinfection with resistant organisms. Migration of the catheters from the infected area is prevented by suturing the tips of the catheters in place with fine absorbable suture. The pump is more likely to flip when the patient is obese and when there is a large amount of fluid in the pump pocket. The only solution is to expose the pump surgically and resuture it to the preabdominal fascia. If a large amount of fluid is present it is cultured. Infection of the pump or catheters is managed with aspiration of the pump pocket and systemic oral antibiotics, when possible. If necessary, the pump is removed and the pocket is closed over a Penrose drain. Systemic antibiotics are administered for 10 days. Superinfection occurs when the wound to which antibiotics are being delivered continues to drain. The most common pathogenic organism is *Candida*. *Candida* infection is suspected when the surrounding soft tissue has a characteristic indurated appearance and dusky cellulitis is present. Cultures of drainage are positive for *Candida* and confirm the diagnosis. In cases in which symptoms are stable, and there are no large retained foreign bodies (eg, a total joint), an oral static agent such as ketoconazole is administered. If symptoms worsen, local antibiotic therapy is discontinued and amphotericin is administered. In cases in which there is a large foreign body present, it is assumed that its surface is colonized with yeast and it will have to be removed to achieve suppression of infection.

Autogenous cancellous bone grafting

The success of cancellous bone grafting techniques are dependent upon the osteoinductive capacity of autogenous cancellous bone. When using these techniques it is important to use only cancellous bone, as cortical bone will become a sequestrum and is not as osteoinductive as cancellous bone. When antibiotics are mixed with the graft, it serves as an antibiotic delivery system, and osteoinduction is not suppressed.[27] The primary limitation of autogenous cancellous grafting is the amount of graft that can be easily obtained. Sources of readily available cancellous bone are the iliac crest, in particular the posterior crest, and the distal femur. More graft can be obtained from the iliac crest than from the distal femur, but there is more postoperative pain following an iliac crest graft. The advantages of obtaining graft from the distal femur are that it is a simple operative exposure, and there is minimal postoperative pain.

In its simplest form, as described by Papineau in the 1970s, morcelized graft is used to fill a granulating defect, which is left open.[1] When granulation tissue grows through the graft, a split thickness skin graft is applied. The advantages of the Papineau technique, or open cancellous grafting, are simplicity and reproducibility. Disadvantages include: extended hospitalization; the large amount of autogenous cancellous bone required; numerous surgical procedures; and the prolonged period of disability while the graft incorporates.[28–30] Certain conditions mitigate against the use of open cancellous grafting. Stable fixation of the affected bone is mandatory and, therefore, segmental defects which cannot be adequately stabilized are not suitable for this technique. Also, the granulation bed into which the bone graft is placed must have a rich vascular supply for graft incorporation. Therefore, this method is not always applicable to chronically infected segmental defects, in which the granulation bed is typically dysvascular. Green and Dlabal reported the results of open cancellous grafting in 15 patients.[31] Stabilization was achieved with external fixation, which was in place an average of 7.5 months. Thirteen of the 15 patients healed their defect, and two underwent amputation.

Calkins et al reported a variation of the Papineau technique in which posttraumatic defects of the upper extremity were filled with a corticocancellous block of iliac crest.[32] The block was inserted into the intercalary defect and stabilized with wires, pins or plates. The wounds were left open and healed secondarily. Sixteen patients were included in the study. None of the ten patients with hand defects developed an infection, but four of the six patients with forearm or arm defects developed an infection. The advantage of using a corticocancellous block of bone instead of morcelized graft was that the graft added stability while filling dead space. The authors conclude that: this method should be limited to subacute reconstruction of posttraumatic defects (i.e., within several weeks of injury); results are better in the hand than the arm and forearm; and that this method should not be used in lower extremity defects.

In its most sophisticated form, cancellous grafting is used in conjunction with a free tissue transfer. PMMA–antibiotic beads are placed underneath the flap to maintain dead space. Three weeks later the beads are removed and autogenous graft is placed in the defect. This "closed cancellous bone grafting" has the advantage of better soft tissue coverage of bone, and requires less strenuous postoperative care than open cancellous grafting. It has the disadvantage of usually requiring a lengthy, technically difficult procedure (free soft tissue transfer). Christian et al were the first to describe this technique and its results clearly in a series of eight patients.[33] All eight patients had sustained a grade IIIB fracture of the tibia and had an average diaphyseal defect 10 cm in length. All eight tibias healed, although one patient developed osteomyelitis. These are remarkable results and argue strongly for the use of this technique in the management of tibial defects. In a further discussion of this technique Bosse and Robb stress the importance of: free tissue transfer; filling the entire bony defect with beads to insure an adequate bone graft column; overlap of the graft with the original diaphysis; and decortication of the surface of the diaphysis to insure that the graft heals to it.[34] Essentially, these authors have followed the basic plan described by Gordon and Chiu by staging the reconstruction of tibial defects (i.e., stage 1 is coverage with a tissue transfer, and stage 2 is bony reconstruction).[15]

An alternative to closed cancellous bone grafting is posterior lateral bone grafting.[35] Posterior lateral bone grafting does not require free soft tissue transfer. In this technique, the nonunion or segmental defect is approached via a posterior lateral exposure. Cancellous graft is placed in the nonunion site or in the segmental gap. Because the bed into which the cancellous bone is placed is very vascular, the graft usually incorporates. In addition, this approach avoids compromised and hypovascular tissue anteriorly. Disadvantages of this technique include: its limited usefulness in the proximal and distal tibia; and the difficulty of performing an adequate débridement, as the surgical approach does not provide adequate exposure for this task.

Technique: iliac crest bone graft

When a large amount of graft is required, the patient is positioned on his or her side or prone. If graft is to be harvested only from the anterior one third of the crest, the patient is positioned supine, with a bolster under the operated side. The skin incision is at the brim of the iliac crest and is carried down to the crest itself. The muscles which attach to the superior aspect of the crest (ie, the internal and external obliques and the erector spinae) are left undisturbed. The periosteum overlying the outer lip of the iliac crest is incised and the gluteus maximus is stripped from the outer table of the ilium using a large periosteal elevator. When stripping the gluteus it is useful to remember that the majority of the cancellous bone is located just under the brim of the ilium, and that the ilium becomes very thin distally; therefore, it is not necessary to strip the muscles off more than the proximal 3 cm of the ilium. The exception to this is posteriorly, where the ilium is thick and there is a large amount of graft along the entire length of the sacroiliac joint. The superior gluteal artery and nerve exit the sciatic notch posteriorly and run anteriorly. To avoid injury to these structures, the exposure of the ilium must be subperiosteal. An osteotome is used to cut the outer cortex of the ilium along its brim. This cut can be extended as far ante-

riorly as the anterior superior iliac spine, and as far posteriorly as the posterior superior iliac spine. Two vertical cuts are now made at the anterior and posterior ends of the horizontal cut. The outer cortex of the ilium is peeled back by undercutting it with a broad osteotome. Cancellous bone is harvested from under the crest with curettes and gouges. If the inner cortex of the ilium is inadvertently windowed, the iliacus muscle protects the structures in the pelvis from injury. When the required cancellous bone has been harvested, the raw bony surfaces are covered with a hemostatic agent, and the outer table of the ilium is pushed back into place. The gluteus maximus is sutured back to the periosteum and fascia of the crest of the ilium, holding the outer table reduced. A suction drain is left in the wound. There are no restrictions postoperatively, but activities are invariably limited by pain for one to three weeks.

Technique: distal femoral bone graft

The patient is positioned supine on the operating table, with a tourniquet around the upper thigh. After the leg has been exsanguinated, and the tourniquet inflated, a midlateral skin incision is made over the lateral femoral condyle. The skin incision extends from the knee joint proximally 4 cm. The fascia lata is divided in line with its fibers, exposing the periosteum of the lateral femoral condyle. The periosteum is incised, and elevated. A half inch osteotome is used to window the cortex 2 cm proximal to the distal articular surface of the femur. Curettes are used to harvest the graft. The defect is filled with an osteoconductive material; I use collagraft (Zimmer, Warsaw, Indiana, USA). The wound is closed in layers without leaving a drain.

Follow up: distal femoral bone graft

Active and passive range of motion of the knee is encouraged postoperatively. Toe touch weight bearing is maintained for one month, after which weight bearing is advanced as tolerated.

Technique: Papineau procedure

The first stage is radical débridement and stabilization of the bone ends. All devitalized and compromised soft tissue and bone are removed. The margins of the wound must be well vascularized and granulate readily. Stabilization is most frequently accomplished with an external fixator. The wound is left open and dressing changes are performed daily until there is a healthy bed of granulation tissue. The defect is then filled with morcelized autogenous cancellous bone. The wound is left open, and the cancellous bone is covered with Vaseline gauze. The first dressing change is at two days, and thereafter at daily intervals. I use a dry dressing with a nonadherent layer applied directly over the graft. Initially the appearance of the wound filled with necrotic cancellous graft is disturbing. However, granulation tissue grows slowly around and through the bone graft. A split thickness skin graft is applied once a layer of granulating tissue covers the graft. Systemic antibiotics are administered until the skin graft is performed.

Follow up: Papineau procedure

Pin care is essential as the external fixator must remain in place until consolidation of the graft has occurred. Weight bearing is not allowed until the graft begins to consolidate. The external fixator is removed only when the defect is healed clinically and radiographically.

Technique: closed bone grafting

This technique is similar to the Papineau technique in that it entails autogenous cancellous grafting of a bony defect. It differs from the Papineau technique in that the site to be grafted must have adequate soft tissue coverage. The first stage is radical débridement, closure of the soft tissue defect with well perfused soft tissue, and stabilization of the bone fragments. Closure is most frequently accomplished with a local rotational muscle flap (gastrocnemius or soleus) or a free flap. Dead space beneath the flap is maintained with PMMA–antibiotic beads. In the second stage, after the wound has healed and the flap has stabilized, the beads are removed and the dead space is filled with autogenous cancellous graft. Removal of the beads is performed as atraumatically as possible to minimize postoperative hematoma. Often, one corner of the flap can be raised, exposing the beads, which are removed. The bed of granulation tissue lining the dead space is gently irrigated of hematoma and the cancellous graft is placed into the defect. Prior to insertion, antibiotics are mixed with the bone graft. I use 1 g vancomycin, 1 g of a second generation cephalosporin, or 1.2 g tobramycin). The wound is closed over the graft.

Follow up: closed bone grafting

In the immediate postoperative period the patient is examined daily for abscess formation. Antibiotics are continued for three weeks from insertion of the bone graft. When the patient is discharged he or she is followed at intervals based on the surgeon's clinical judgment. Weight bearing is not allowed until the graft has consolidated.

Technique: posterolateral bone grafting

The patient is positioned prone, with a tourniquet around the thigh. A cancellous graft is harvested from the posterior iliac crest. This wound is then closed and covered. The tourniquet is inflated and a longitudinal incision is made parallel with, and 1 cm posterior to, the posterior border of the fibula. The interval between the triceps surae and the peroneals is developed.

The peroneals are retracted anteriorly and the gastrocnemius and soleus posteriorly, exposing the fibula. The dissection is carried around the posterior surface of the fibula to the interosseous membrane. Here the posterior tibialis is stripped from the interosseous membrane and posterior surface of the tibia. The posterior tibial artery and nerve are located between the posterior tibial muscle and the soleus. Therefore, the artery and nerve are not at risk if the posterior tibial muscle is identified and elevated from its origin on the tibia and interosseous membrane. The cortex of the tibia, proximal and distal to the nonunion, is decorticated with an osteotome, and the autogenous bone graft, mixed with antibiotic, is placed in the nonunion site. The wound is closed over a drain. In cases which are actively infected, stabilization is best achieved with an external fixator. Casting, plating and intramedullary nailing have also been described as methods of stabilization.

Follow up: posterolateral bone grafting

In the immediate postoperative period the patient is carefully monitored for signs of abscess formation. If these signs are present, the graft site is débrided as they emerge. In cases which are actively infected, systemic antibiotics are initiated at the time of surgery and are continued for a minimum of three weeks. In cases with a quiescent infection, the antibiotics may be discontinued when the patient is discharged from the hospital (usually after four to seven days). Weight bearing depends upon the method of stabilization and the inherent stability of the nonunion.

External fixation

The advantage of external fixation in the management of infected fractures and nonunions is that stabilization is achieved without introducing a large foreign body into an infected wound and without an extensive surgical approach. In the past, external fixation was static (ie, once the frame had been applied, the fracture fragments could not be moved) and was limited to fractures and nonunions of the diaphysis. Now, dynamic external fixators allow manipulation of bone segments and small wire circular frame external fixators have expanded the indications to periarticular and even intraarticular fractures and nonunions. Dynamic external fixators can be used to compress or distract fractures and nonunions, and therefore are used not only for stabilization, but also to achieve bony consolidation or to form new bone through the process of distraction osteogenesis. The disadvantages of external fixation are that patient acceptance is frequently limited, and pin tracts may become infected.

Static external fixation

Static external fixation is used to immobilize bone segments. By itself, static external fixation will not result in consolidation of a nonunion or filling in of a defect. Therefore, it is always combined with other procedures when it is used in the management of nonunions or segmental defects (eg, autogenous cancellous grafting, or vascularized bone segment transfer).

Uniplanar frames are smaller and better tolerated by the patient than circular frames. Uniplanar frames depend upon the stiffness of pins, which are fixed to bone with threads, to transmit stresses to the fixator. One of the major advantages of uniplanar frames is that transfixion of muscles and other soft tissue is minimized. Circular frames depend upon tensioned small diameter wires, which are fastened to the fixator for stability. Wire orientation and spacing is key to maximize stability. The wires are oriented nearly 90° to each other and spaced above and below the circular frame. Circular frames are of value in the management of intraarticular and periarticular nonunions.

Their major disadvantage is that more soft tissue is transfixed by pins than when a unilateral frame is used.

Technique: static external fixation

The key to the successful application of an external fixator is the location of the pins and the technique with which the pins are inserted into the bone. The pins should be located in healthy bone, away from the site of the infection. To minimize the risk to nerves and arteries during pin insertion, pins are inserted via "safe zones", or areas in which there are no major nerves or arteries. When it is not feasible to insert a pin via a safe zone, nerves or arteries at risk are exposed surgically and retracted out of harm's way. Surgical exposure of a neurovascular structure at risk is most frequently necessary when applying a lateral fixator to the humerus (radial nerve) or a dorsal fixator to the distal radius (superficial radial nerve). Ideally, the pins should not violate muscles or tendons. Therefore, when applying the fixator to the tibia, half pins are inserted from the anteromedial side of the tibia. In cases in which a pin must be inserted through a muscle, the pin is inserted when the muscle is stretched to its maximum length (eg: when inserting a lateral frame on the femur, the vastus lateralis is stretched by flexing the knee; when inserting a pin through the peroneal muscles, the ankle is plantar flexed and the foot supinated; and when inserting a pin through the anterior tibial muscle, the ankle is plantar flexed).

When the optimum location has been determined, the pin is inserted into the bone. It is important to cause as little tissue necrosis as possible when inserting the pin. Therefore, skin and soft tissue overlying the bone are incised down to the bone. Simply incising the skin and pushing the pin through overlying tissue to the bone is poor technique. If a large diameter pin is being used, the bone is predrilled to minimize heat necrosis. Tissue protecting sleeves are utilized during the drilling and insertion of the pins. At the conclusion of external fixator application, all pin sites are examined to determine whether any of the pins are exerting tension on overlying soft tissue. If they are, releases are performed by incising the soft tissue, or the pins are removed and replaced.

Follow up: static external fixation

Weight bearing and the length of time that the fixator is maintained are tailored to each case. Follow up care is designed to prolong the life of the fixator by minimizing pin tract complications. The patient is instructed to keep the pin sites scrupulously clean. Cotton swabs are used to remove debris from around the pins twice a day. Rinsing the fixator in clean tap water once a day is encouraged. When pin sites become inflamed, there are five possible courses of action: release the pin sites using local anesthesia and a scalpel; reemphasize the importance of maintaining the cleanliness of the fixator; prescribe whirlpool therapy to insure cleanliness; administer broad spectrum oral antibiotics; and, as a last resort, remove the pins. In cases in which the pins are removed because of inflammation, the pin site should be managed as a focus of osteomyelitis, ie, necrotic bone and soft tissue are débrided by curetting the pin tract and the wound is packed open. Systemic antibiotics are administered for four to six weeks. The antibiotic administered is determined by the pathogenic organisms and their sensitivities. This information is obtained by culturing material obtained at the surgical débridement.

Dynamic external fixation

Dynamic external fixators are used to compress and distract nonunions, to promote healing, and to form bone via distraction osteogenesis.

The concept of dynamic external fixation has been in existence since the early twentieth century. Putti and then Abbott described external fixators which were used to gradually lengthen the femur and tibia respectively through complex geometric osteotomies.[36,37] Both Putti and Abbott attributed the majority of the success of their techniques to the shape of the osteotomy, and not to callus distraction or distraction osteogenesis. Yet, the radiographic appearance of the lengthened tibia in Abbott's paper is identical to that of a tibia lengthened with modern techniques. Enthusiasm for this early technique of dynamic external fixation was never overwhelming, in Abbott's case primarily because of the amount of pain that the patients experienced during the lengthening (P. M. Manske and D.O. Burst, personal communications). Dynamic external fixation was abandoned until a Russian, Gavriel Ilizarov, rediscovered it in the 1950s. Ilizarov is credited with originating the modern technique of distraction osteogenesis achieved with dynamic external fixation. He used this technique to manage a variety of conditions affecting the extremities, including segmental defects. The success of distraction osteogenesis is dependent upon osteogenesis, which occurs during distraction of an osteotomy site. To accomplish this, the cortex of the involved bone is cut circumferentially at a site distant to the segmental defect; the resulting free segment of bone is distracted and transported slowly within its periosteal sleeve through the segmental defect to the nonunion docking site. Stimulated by this distraction, regenerate bone forms in the osteotomy site. It is the *de novo* formation of bone which makes distraction osteogenesis unique. The advantages of distraction osteogenesis are that: large autogenous bone grafts are unnecessary; and early weight bearing is encouraged. In addition, angiogenesis of small vessels may be stimulated, thus increasing local blood flow. The disadvantages include: the need for exceptional patient compliance and tolerance; frame application is a technically difficult procedure with an extended learning curve; and finally, patients must be followed closely and the frame adjusted frequently.

Dynamic external fixation is achieved using one of two basic types of fixators: a large pin unilateral frame or a small wire circular frame. The large pin unilateral frame is used when no angular correction is required (ie, simple unipolar lengthening); it is less bulky than equivalent small wire circular frames. Large pin unilateral frames have a lower profile and are better tolerated by the patient. The small wire circular frames are used in cases in which there is angular or translational deformity and when there is a periarticular nonunion or malunion. Because large pin frames are considered to be more "user friendly", they are often combined with small wire circular frames to form a "hybrid" frame. Hybrid frames consist of a periarticular circular small wire ring fastened to a diaphyseal large pin frame.

As the technique of distraction osteogenesis is relatively new, there is a dearth of large long term series which have been published in peer reviewed journals. Therefore, it is difficult to compare the results obtained using distraction osteogenesis with those obtained using other methods. Tucker et al reported seven cases in which there was a segmental defect of the tibia or in which the tibia had been shortened.[38] A small wire circular frame was used to manage the defect or shortening, which averaged about 4 cm in length. The number of surgical procedures requiring general anesthesia averaged 2.5, and attests to the expected rate of complications. Two patients refractured, one developed chronic osteomyelitis at a pin tract, and two patients had equinus contractures of the ankle. Paley et al reported a larger series, 25 patients, with nonunions of the tibia treated with small wire circular frames.[39,40] This was a diverse group of patients: 13 were actively infected; 22 nonunions were atrophic, 3 were hypertrophic; 12 had a segmental defect, and 13 had a deformity. Although it is difficult to analyze results from such a diverse group, it is clear that these patients all had severe problems, and as expected there was a high incidence of complications, which ranged in severity from sympathetic dystrophy to amputation for neurogenic pain. The authors conclude that "The ability to achieve an excellent bony result in even the worst of bony pathologic conditions does not guarantee a good functional result unless the patient has an acceptable neurovascular status."

As experience with distraction osteogenesis has accumulated in Western Europe and North America, it has been possible to make several generalizations. The production of regenerate bone during the technique of distraction osteogenesis is a reliable phenomena. Major complications are common and include psychological intolerance of the frame and failure to obtain union of the transported segment at the "docking site". Minor complications such as pin breakage, pin tract infection, joint stiffness and premature consolidation of the regenerate bone are also common, but their occurrence does not preclude a good result. The lowest incidence of complications occurs when the technique is used for tibial defects; the highest incidence of complications occurs when it is used in the management of femoral defects.

Technique: dynamic external fixation

Patient selection and education are extremely important. A history of mental disorders or substance abuse is a contraindication to this technique.[41,42] The ideal patient is motivated and stoic. The patient must understand what the technique entails and the necessity of his or her cooperation for success. Constructing the frame and showing it to the patient prior to its application increases patient compliance.

The goals of treatment are defined as one or more of the following: lengthening; consolidation of a nonunion; correction of angular deformity; or correction of translational deformity. Usually the tibia is involved; occasionally the femur or humerus are involved. Based upon these goals the frame is designed and fabricated preoperatively.

When the goal of therapy is lengthening alone, I use a "track and trolley" large pin unilateral frame (Fig. 6.12). Frame design is simple. The frame must be large enough to accommodate the planned lengthening. When the goal of therapy is consolidation of a nonunion without correction of deformity or lengthening, a "ball

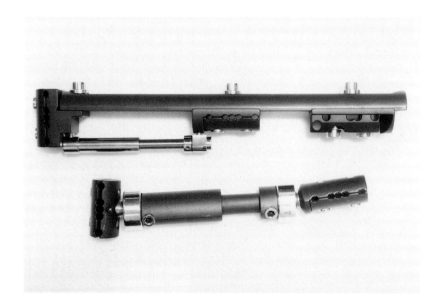

Figure 6.12

A "track and trolley" large pin external fixator used for the management of segmental defects or lengthening, and a "ball joint" external fixator used for the management of nonunions.

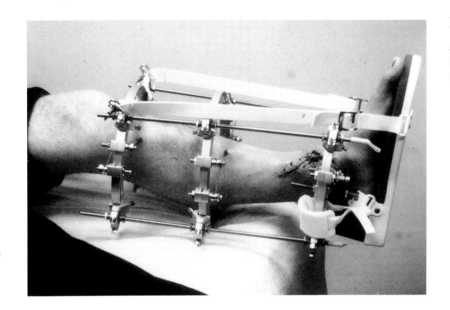

Figure 6.13

A small wire circular frame used for the correction of angular deformity.

joint" large pin unilateral frame is used (Fig. 6.12). When the goal of therapy is lengthening and consolidation of a nonunion without correction of deformity, a "track and trolley" large pin unilateral frame is used. A minimum of three clamps are always required. When lengthening is via two corticotomies four clamps are used. When the goal of therapy is correction of angular and translational deformity, a small wire circular frame is used, as large pin unilateral frames with hinges have not been available until recently (Fig. 6.13). As experience is gained with large pin frames that are able to correct translational rotational and angular deformities, these frames may supplant small wire circular frames.

The following is a description of small wire circular tibial frame design, but the principles can be applied to the femur or humerus. The first step is to determine the plane and magnitude of the deformity. The angular deformity is measured on anteroposterior and lateral radiographs. It is essential that the projection of the radiographs be reproducible because they will determine the position of the frame during surgery (Fig. 6.14). The angles are plotted to deter-

mine the exact plane and magnitude of the deformity (Fig. 6.15). The second step is construction of the frame to correct the deformity. Rings are positioned parallel with the knee and ankle and at right angles to the long axis of the segment of the diaphysis. Hinges are placed over the apex of the deformity and at right angles to it. The apex of deformity is defined as the intersection point of the lines drawn down the center of each diaphyseal segment, parallel with the long axis of the segment. When only angular deformity is present, the apex of deformity is directly over the site of the nonunion. When there is angular and translational deformity, the apex is proximal or distal to the site of the nonunion.

The first stage of the surgical procedure is application of the external fixator to the extremity. Pin placement is chosen to minimize the chance of neurovascular damage and to avoid tendons and nerves. When a monolateral half frame is utilized this is fairly simple; the full pins used with small wire circular frames makes avoidance of these structures more difficult. The rings of a small wire circular fixator are

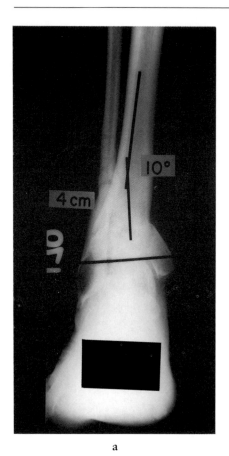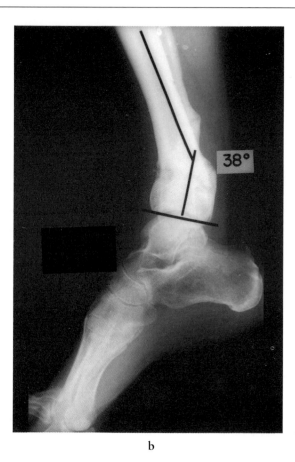

a   b

Figure 6.14

Radiographs in the anteroposterior (a) and lateral (b) projections of an ankle. Clinically the patient has a non-union of the distal tibia. The fibula is healed. The angles of deformity in these projections are 10° and 38° respectively. In addition there is 4 cm of shortening.

positioned in such a way that when the rings are parallel with each other the deformity is corrected. In the correction of a deformity of the distal tibia, the distal ring is in the plane of the ankle mortise, and the proximal rings are positioned at right angles to the diaphysis (Fig. 6.16).

The second stage of the procedure is osteotomy. Prior to osteotomy the wires or pins are drilled into the segment of bone that will be osteotomized. The cortex of the involved bone is cut circumferentially with as little damage to the periosteum and medullary contents as possible. Because only the cortex is cut, this osteotomy is more specifically called a corticotomy. The corticotomy is usually performed in the metaphyseal region of the involved bone. In the tibia, a longitudinal incision is made over the crest of the tibia, exposing the periosteum. The periosteum is incised and carefully elevated. A one quarter inch osteotome is used to cut medial and lateral cortices. Every effort is made to pro-

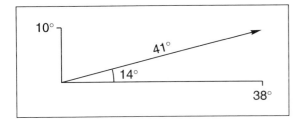

Figure 6.15

The angles derived from the radiographs are the result of the true deformity, the magnitude and direction of which are as yet undetermined. To determine the parameters of the true deformity, the angles derived from the radiographs are plotted. The resultant indicates the magnitude and direction of the true deformity, in this case the deformity is in a plane 14° from the sagittal plane and has a magnitude of 41°.

tect the medullary contents and the periosteum. The corticotomy is completed through the posterior cortex of the tibia by twisting the osteotome or by loosening the frame and using it gently to twist the tibia. A free segment of bone which is connected to the frame by half pins or

wires has been produced by the corticotomy. One to two weeks after the corticotomy, transportation of the free segment begins. The transported segment of bone is transported at a rate of 0.5 mm to 1 mm per day, in 0.25 mm increments. The rate and rhythm of distraction can be varied according to the patient's profile (eg, age, nutritional status, and clinical response).

Several variations of this technique have been described. Two corticotomies can be performed in the same bone, one distal and one proximal to the segmental nonunion. With two transported segments of bone, the time period of treatment is shortened by about 25%. Another variation is acute shortening of the tibia by approximating the nonunion fragments. Leg lengthening is then performed using distraction osteogenesis. The nonunion is sequentially compressed and distracted during the lengthening and consolidation of the corticotomy.

Follow up: dynamic external fixation

The surgical procedure is technically demanding but straightforward. The follow up is challenging

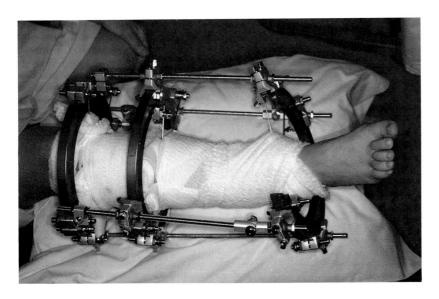

Figure 6.16

The frame is constructed with hinges in the plane of the true deformity, and in such a way that when the rings are parallel, the deformity will be corrected; in this case the distal ring is parallel to the plane of the ankle mortise, and the proximal rings are at right angles to the tibial diaphysis. In order to correct the deformity through the nonunion the fibula is osteotomized. To obtain the 4 cm of length, a corticotomy has been performed between the two proximal rings.

and frequently frustrating. Patients are usually discharged one to four days following frame application and corticotomy. Pin care is extremely important as the frame will be in place for months. At seven days to two weeks after corticotomy, distraction is begun at the corticotomy site at a rate of 0.5 mm–1 mm a day. The patient is followed weekly for at least one month and then biweekly. At each follow up, radiographs are obtained to evaluate distraction, regenerate bone formation, and frame position. If distraction is not occurring, the corticotomy may have to be redone. Regenerate bone should appear about four weeks following the corticotomy. If it has not appeared by six weeks, distraction should be stopped or temporarily reversed. The patient is carefully monitored for pin tract infections, weight bearing status, and development of joint contractures. Pin tract infections are treated with systemic or local antibiotics, whirlpool and, if necessary, by changing the pins. If weight bearing decreases or contractures develop, the rate of distraction is slowed and rigorous physical therapy initiated. If the contractures do not resolve, surgical releases may have to be performed if further correction of deformity or lengthening is required (Fig. 6.17). In our experience all patients treated with this method have significant pain and require analgesics during therapy. External fixation is maintained until the regenerate bone has consolidated and matured, as indicated by the appearance of cortical bone. Dynamization of the frame may accelerate this process. Typically, the external fixator is maintained for a total period of time roughly equal to three times the distraction period.

The complications of dynamic external fixation are: failure of the frame (eg, pin breakage); joint contracture; joint subluxation; spontaneous arthrodesis; loss of correction following frame removal; and failure of consolidation at the docking site. Management of frame failure is frame revision (Fig. 6.18). Management of contractures, subluxation or arthrodesis (Fig. 6.19) is: early recognition of loss of motion; decreasing the rate of lengthening; and institution of physi-

cal therapy. Loss of correction following removal of the frame is managed with casting and nonweight bearing until the regenerate bone has matured further, or application of a second frame. Failure of consolidation at the docking site is managed by internal fixation of the nonunion with a plate or nail and bone grafting (Fig. 6.20).

Internal fixation

The achievement of stability of associated fractures and nonunions is an integral part of the management of osteomyelitis. When external fixation is not an option, plates or intramedullary nails are used to achieve stability. Regardless of how stability is achieved, we must also consider how to stimulate the fracture or nonunion to heal. In general, hypertrophic nonunions only require stability as a stimulus to consolidate. Fractures and atrophic nonunions are bone grafted.

Plates

The use of plates to reestablish bony continuity has several advantages: fixation is rigid, and therefore surrounding joints can be mobilized; and malalignment associated with the nonunion can be accurately corrected under direct vision. Burri stated that the advantages of plate stabilization of infected nonunions were that plating "has a favorable effect on the infectious component, accelerates the consolidation of the bone which may be spontaneous or induced, and in addition permits active physical therapy".[43] However, he cautioned that plate osteosynthesis must result in absolute stability, be via a surgical approach through healthy tissue, and that the plate must be covered by live tissue (muscle if possible).

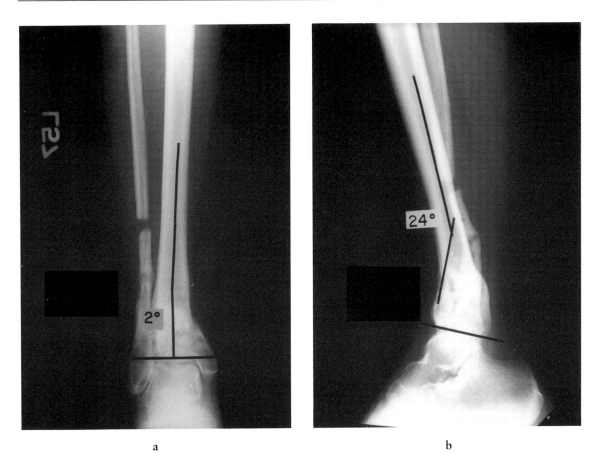

a   b

Figure 6.17

Postframe removal the deformity has been corrected to 2° and 24° as seen on the anteroposterior (a) and lateral (b) radiographs. Further correction of the angular deformity was not possible as the patient had a longstanding equinus contracture of the foot which became clinically increasingly evident.

Helfet et al reported the results of plating 33 tibial nonunions, 16 of which had latent osteo-myelitis.[44] All nonunions consolidated, and only one patient developed a postoperative infection. This patient had latent osteomyelitis. The authors conclude that the risk of activating latent osteomyelitis is not a contraindication to plating of a tibial nonunion. Several details of the authors' technique explain their astoundingly good results: all nonunions were grafted with autogenous cancellous bone; the plate was placed

on the tension side of the bone; a lag screw was used whenever possible; and, perhaps most importantly, indirect reduction with a femoral distracter minimized the dissection.

Wiss et al reported less favorable results in a similar series, of 50 nonunions of the tibia, which were plated following initial management with external fixation.[45] The main thrust of this paper was to determine whether plating was a safe procedure following external fixation. The surgical technique used by Wiss et al was similar

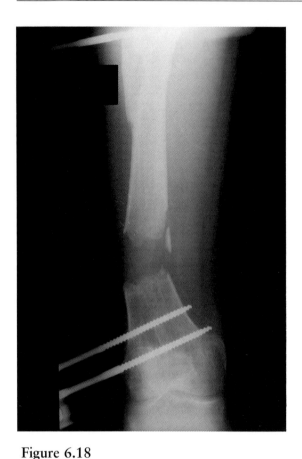

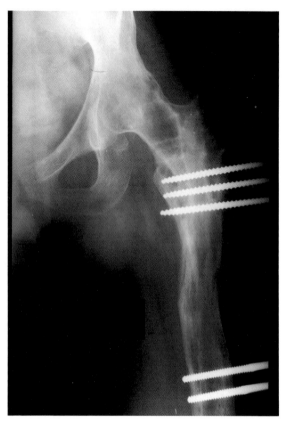

Figure 6.18

Failure of a "ball joint" frame during femoral lengthening has resulted in loss of alignment. Because of this type of failure, I no longer use "ball joint" type fixators for lengthening. Instead I use the "track and trolley" type fixator.

Figure 6.19

Spontaneous ankylosis of the hip joint during lengthening of the femur.

to that of Helfet et al, in that indirect reduction was used to minimize dissection, the plate was applied to the tension side of the tibia, and only atrophic nonunions were bone grafted. In the series reported by Wiss et al, 46 of the 50 nonunions consolidated. Five patients had a clear history of osteomyelitis (ie, drainage from the fracture or a pin site) but had been asymptomatic for a minimum of ten weeks prior to plating. Three of these five patients developed an

infection. In two the infection resolved with intravenous antibiotics alone; in the third patient the plate broke, and was removed. The authors conclude that nonunions with a history of infection should be biopsied, and that culture positive biopsies are a contraindication to plating. The disparity between these papers is not easily explained, although my experience has been closer to that reported by Wiss et al.

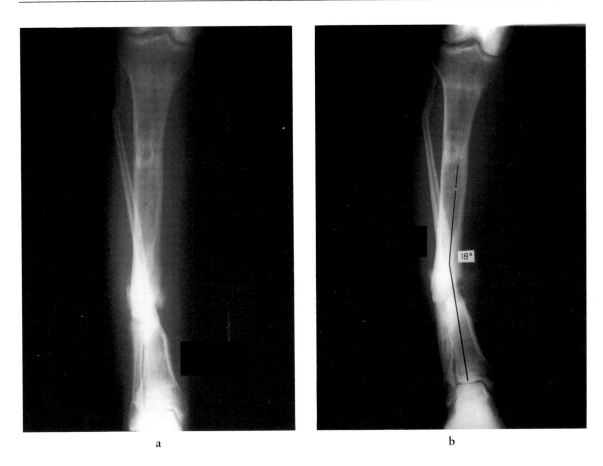

a   b

Figure 6.20

Radiograph of a tibia following frame removal. A segmental defect has been managed with bone transport. The docking site is 7 cm proximal to the ankle; the corticotomy site is 7 cm distal to the knee (a). Clinically the docking site was healed; however, a deformity developed over the next six months (b). The unhealed docking site was managed with correction of the deformity and intramedullary nailing.

The disadvantages of using plates to reestablish bony continuity in the presence of infection are: the possibility of exacerbation of infection due to the extensive dissection necessary to position the plate; the plate is a foreign body and may become a source of persistent infection; and, as the plate is load bearing, there is a high incidence of failure of fixation. Plate osteosynthesis is a particularly good way to manage periarticular and intraarticular nonunions. Juxtaarticular fragments of bone are frequently best held in place with buttress plates and interfragmental screws.

Technique: plates

The technique of plate osteosynthesis of infected fractures, delayed unions, and nonunions is broken down into three stages: surgical exposure;

correction of associated deformity; and application of the plate.

The surgical exposure is the key to success. The exposure is designed to minimize the chance of tissue necrosis in an area that is frequently at increased risk because of prior surgical procedures and the presence of infection. Therefore, the skin incision is through scars from previous incisions; flaps are not raised unless absolutely necessary. If a flap is raised, it should be thick, if possible consisting of skin subcutaneous tissue and periosteum. In cases in which there is a hypertrophic nonunion, the flap can also include bone.

When adequate exposure of the nonunion has been achieved, any associated malalignment is corrected. This is most frequently accomplished by "taking down" the nonunion, ie, the removal and lysis of fibrous tissue between the unhealed bone ends. Occasionally a malaligned nonunion is left in situ, and a corrective osteotomy is performed proximally or distally. This technique is useful in the management of hypertrophic periarticular nonunions in which there is limited room for fixation. The osteotomy is located so that the nonunion is between it and the joint, allowing the hypertrophic bone about the nonunion to be used as a point of fixation. In the specific case of a malaligned tibial nonunion, the fibula must be osteotomized if it has healed, prior to correcting the malalignment of the tibia. The fibular osteotomy is performed through a second incision if necessary, and is located at least 10 cm distal to the head of the fibula (to avoid injury of the common peroneal nerve), and 6 cm proximal to the ankle joint (to avoid destabilizing the ankle joint). Locating the fibular osteotomy at the level of the nonunion facilitates correction of malalignment, but may eliminate the possibility of other procedures, such as posterior lateral bone graft and Huntington fibular transfer, in the future.

Plate application is straightforward. In general, larger plates are used for the osteosynthesis of infected nonunions than for fresh fractures (eg, a large fragment broad dynamic compression plate is used for the tibia). Cancellous and cortical screws are utilized according to the judgment of the surgeon.

Follow up: plates

Postoperatively, the patient is carefully observed for abscess or hematoma formation. Antibiotics are administered until the postoperative swelling and cellulitis has resolved. When an actively infected fracture or nonunion has been plated we administer systemic antibiotics for three to six weeks. Our rationale is that antibiotics inhibit bacterial colonization of the plate, and diminish the chance of raging postoperative infections. When the antibiotics are discontinued, the patient is carefully observed for recurrent abscess formation. Draining sinuses and ulcers are managed with local wound care.

Physical therapy and activity level are the keys to success. Active range of motion exercises are encouraged to maintain and increase motion through neighboring joints. Passive motion and weight bearing are not allowed until there is clear radiographic evidence of healing, ie, trabeculae which cross the nonunion or fracture. There are two mistakes which are frequently made in the postoperative management. The first is immobilization of the extremity in an effort to protect the plate osteosynthesis. This results in loss of motion of neighboring joints, resulting in an increase in the length of the lever arm through the nonunion and a high incidence of failure of fixation. The second mistake made in postoperative management is premature passive motion or weight bearing, resulting in failure of fixation. This mistake is made because after the incisional pain subsides, the patient feels as though the fracture or nonunion has healed. With rigid plate fixation there is no sensation of movement between fragments of bone until the fixation fails.

Following consolidation of the fracture or nonunion, regardless of whether the patient has latent or active osteomyelitis, the plate and screws are removed and the wound is débrided (necrotic bone is frequently found beneath the plate), and if the patient is still actively infected a second course of antibiotics is administered.

Intramedullary nails

Intramedullary nailing is an excellent way to manage aseptic nonunions of the tibia and femur.[46,47] It is not a good way to manage nonunions of the humerus. Foster et al reported a series of humeral fractures and nonunions which were stabilized in various ways.[48] They found that Kuntscher nails resulted in consolidation in only 8 of 11 nonunions and that there was a high incidence of impingement on the rotator cuff.

The place of intramedullary nailing in the management tibial or femoral nonunions with latent osteomyelitis is less firmly established than it is with aseptic nonunions. The major disadvantage is that this technique risks exacerbating or activating the infection. Galpin et al reported a series of 18 patients with nonunions of the tibia secondary to failed plating managed with removal of the plate and reamed intramedullary nailing.[49] Sixteen of the 18 healed their nonunion. Among the 18 patients there were two with a history of infection and one who was actively infected. These three patients developed a postoperative infection, one of which remained active until the patient died from unrelated causes. The authors conclude that although a high rate of union is obtained, this technique "should be considered primarily for uninfected patients".

Fischer et al reported similar poor results with reamed intramedullary nailing in the presence of latent osteomyelitis.[50] In their series of 43 patients who had sustained grade IIIB fractures of the tibia, 19 underwent delayed reamed nailing an average of 27 weeks after injury. None of these fractures were actively infected at the time of nailing; however, all but one had been initially managed with an external fixator. The external

fixator had been removed an average of 13 weeks prior to nailing. Ten patients went on to consolidate their nonunions, but nine developed deep infections. Only two of these nine patients healed their nonunion.

My results were similar in a series of 18 patients with tibial nonunions and latent osteomyelitis managed with reamed intramedullary nails.[51] These 18 patients had a definite history of osteomyelitis but no signs of infection at the time of nailing. All 18 patients underwent surgical biopsy at least two weeks after antibiotics had been discontinued and two weeks prior to nailing. In four cases organisms were cultured from the biopsy material. In 17 cases reamings were sent for culture prior to administration of antibiotics during the intramedullary nailing. Intraoperative cultures were negative in 11 cases and positive in 6. Bacteriologic studies are shown in Table 6.1. Ten patients developed signs of postoperative infection with culture positive drainage. Eleven of the 18 patients healed their nonunion and have no signs of active infection. However, of these 11 patients only 5 healed uneventfully with no signs of infection during their recovery. In seven patients the nonunion did not consolidate. Two of these patients underwent below knee amputation. Based upon my series and those of Galpin et al and Fischer et al, I conclude that a history of infection is a relative contraindication to a reamed intramedullary nail. The major risk is activating a latent infection. It is also clear that a negative preoperative and intraoperative biopsy does not rule out the possibility of exacerbating the infection; however a positive surgical biopsy and positive intraoperative culture indicates an increased chance of exacerbating the infection. Therefore, two questions remain regarding nailing of nonunions with latent osteomyelitis. (1) Could the incidence of activation of infection be minimized by prolonged postoperative administration of local or systemic antibiotics? (2) Should the procedure be done in two stages – reaming and culturing followed by nailing of culture negative patients?

Table 6.1   Culture results from 18 patients with tibial nonunions and latent osteomyelitis

Patient	Original cultures	Biopsy	Intraoperative	Postoperative	Flare up	Final result
1	*Enterobacter cloacae*	Negative	Negative	*Enterobacter cloacae*	Yes	Nail removed after consolidation. Systemic antibiotics for 4 weeks. No signs of active infection
2	*Acinetobacter anitratus*	Negative	Not done	None	No	Nail removed. Small wire circular frame external fixator applied
3	*E. coli*	Negative	Negative	*E. coli*	Yes	Nail removed after consolidation. Systemic antibiotics for 4 weeks. No signs of active infection
4	*S. aureus*	Negative	Negative	None	No	Nonunion consolidated uneventfully
5	*S. epidermidis*	Negative	Negative	No growth	Yes	Nail left in place. Incision and drainage of sterile abscess. Nonunion healed
6	Methicillin-resistant *S. aureus*	Negative	Methicillin-resistant *S. aureus*	Methicillin-resistant *S. aureus*	Yes	Nail removed to control infection. Small wire circular frame external fixator applied
7	*S. aureus*	Negative	*S. epidermidis*	None	No	Nonunion consolidated uneventfully
8	Methicillin-resistant *S. aureus*	Methicillin-resistant *S. aureus*	Methicillin-resistant *S. aureus*	Methicillin-resistant *S. aureus*	Yes	Nail removed after consolidation. Antibiotics for 6 weeks. No signs of active infection
9	Methicillin-resistant *S. epidermidis*	Methicillin-resistant *S. epidermidis*	Negative	None	No	Nail fractured. Renailed

Table 6.1   (contd)

Patient	Original cultures	Biopsy	Intraoperative	Postoperative	Flare up	Final result
10	Methicillin-resistant S. epidermidis	Methicillin-resistant S. epidermidis	Negative	Methicillin-resistant S. epidermidis	Yes	Nail removed after consolidation. Antibiotics for 6 weeks. No signs of active infection
11	Streptococcus S. aureus Enterobacter cloacae Pseudomonas aeruginosa	Negative	Negative	S. aureus Pseudomonas aeruginosa	Yes	Nail removed to control infection. Small wire circular frame external fixator applied
12	S. aureus	Negative	Negative	Negative	No	Nonunion consolidated uneventually
13	S. aureus	Negative	S. aureus	S. aureus	Yes	Below knee amputation to control infection
14	S. aureus	Negative	S. aureus	S. aureus	Yes	Nail left in place. Signs of infection disappeared following consolidation of nonunion
15	Methicillin-resistant S. epidermidis	Methicillin-resistant S. epidermidis	Methicillin-resistant S. epidermidis	Methicillin-resistant S. epidermidis Peptococcus magnus	Yes	Below knee amputation to control infection
16	S. aureus	Negative	Negative	Negative	No	Nonunion consolidated uneventfully
17	Pseudomonas aeruginosa Bacillus subtilis	Negative	Negative	None	No	Nonunion consolidated uneventfully
18	Enterobacter cloacae S. aureus Streptococcus	Negative	Negative	S. aureus	Yes	Persistent nonunion. Small wire circular frame external fixator applied

Stabilization of nonunions which are actively infected with intramedullary nails is controversial. Sledge et al reported the results of reamed intramedullary nailing of 54 tibial nonunions.[52] Among these 54 were eight nonunions which were actively infected at the time of nailing. Following nailing, three of the eight had persistent drainage, and two of these three nonunions did not consolidate. The authors conclude that infection increases "the danger of complications" and that intramedullary nailing of an infected tibial nonunion should be considered a last resort.

My experience with reamed intramedullary nails in the management of infected tibial nonunions has been similar to that of Sledge et al. I managed 16 patients with 17 actively infected tibial nonunions with reamed intramedullary nailing and local administration of the antibiotic amikacin via an implanted pump.[53] The mean duration of symptoms was three years. All 16 patients had previously been treated unsuccessfully surgically at least twice and had received a minimum of four consecutive weeks of intravenous antibiotics at least once. Two patients have been lost to follow up, leaving 14 patients with 15 infected nonunions. Systemic levels of aminoglycoside were determined at seven day intervals during therapy and were always less than half the recommended trough level. Pre- and posttherapy audiograms and creatine clearances (CrCls) documented that there was no eighth nerve toxicity and only one case of subclinical nephrotoxicity. One patient's CrCl dropped to 55 ml/min (70 ml/min is the lower limit of normal). In all 15 nonunions, drainage slowly decreased and stopped during antibiotic administration. Ten patients remained free of signs of infection. Five patients began to drain or developed cellulitis after antibiotics were discontinued. Thirteen nonunions healed. The two patients whose nonunions did not heal also had recurrent infection and underwent below knee amputation. Complications included: injury of the posterior tibial artery and two pump site infections necessitating pump removal and administration of systemic antibiotics. Based on my series and that of Sledge et al, I conclude that reamed intramedullary nailing of an actively infected tibial nonunion should only be undertaken as a last resort. It should be combined with prolonged administration of antibiotics.

Technique: reamed intramedullary nails

The procedure can be performed on a fracture table or with the extremity draped "free" on a radiolucent table. The fracture table facilitates distal locking. Draping the extremity free facilitates correction of deformity and removal of hardware. The nonunion is nailed with a closed technique if possible, but frequently it is necessary to take down the nonunion to correct translational and angular deformity. Osteotomy of the fibula may be necessary to correct the deformity. When it is necessary to open the nonunion, soft tissue stripping of the bone ends is avoided. If a pump is being used to deliver antibiotics locally, the outflow catheters of the pump are led subcutaneously down the thigh, and either are inserted down the lumen of the nail to a point just distal to the area of the nonunion, or they are tunneled subcutaneously to the infected area and placed to give the best spread of antibiotic. If the catheters are inserted down the lumen of the nail, an open section nail is used and the nail cannot be locked proximally. A flexible bronchial biopsy forceps is used to insert the catheters down the lumen of the nail.

Follow up: reamed intramedullary nails

Postoperatively, weight bearing and nail dynamization is tailored to each patient. The nail is removed when the nonunion has consolidated. In cases in which a pump has been implanted, serum levels of aminoglycoside and creatinine confirm the absence of toxicity. Intravenous antibiotics are continued for a minimum of five doses to protect the pump site from infection. The pump is refilled percutaneously as an outpatient procedure.

Complications: reamed intramedullary nails

Complications include: loss of fixation; flare up of infection; pump site infection. Loss of fixation is frequently accompanied by persistent infection. If possible the fixation is revised to stabilize the nonunion. If revision is not possible, an external fixator is applied. Occasionally amputation is the only course of action possible. Flare up of infection is managed with incision, drainage, débridement. The nail is not removed if it is stabilizing the nonunion. In cases in which fixation has been lost, a fixator is applied. Material is sent for culture to rule out a change in the identity or sensitivities of the pathogenic organisms.

References

1 Papineau LJ, L'excision-greffe avec fermeture retardée deliberée dans l'osteomyelite chronique, *Nouv Presse Med* (1973) 2:2753.

2 Knight MP, Wood GO, Surgical obliteration of bone cavities following traumatic osteomyelitis, *J Bone Joint Surg* (1945) 27:547–556.

3 Kelly RP, Rosati LM, Murray RA, Traumatic osteomyelitis. The use of skin grafts, Part 1: technic and results, *Ann Surg* (1945) 122:1–11.

4 Evans ME, Davies DM, The treatment of chronic osteomyelitis by saucerisation and secondary skin grafting, *J Bone Joint Surg* (1969) 51B:454–457.

5 Gupta RC, Treatment of chronic osteomyelitis by radical excision of bone and secondary skin-grafting, *J Bone Joint Surg* (1973) 55A:371–374.

6 Ger R, Efron G, New operative approach in the treatment of chronic osteomyelitis of the tibial diaphysis: a preliminary report, *Clin Orthop Rel Res* (1970) 70:160–169.

7 Ger R, Muscle transposition for treatment and prevention of chronic post-traumatic osteomyelitis of the tibia, *J Bone Joint Surg* (1977) 59A:784–791.

8 Stern PJ, Carey JP, The latissimus dorsi flap for reconstruction of the brachium and shoulder, *J Bone Joint Surg* (1988) 70A:526–535.

9 Salibian AH, Anzel SH, Rogers FR, The gluteus medius tensor fasciae latae myocutaneous flap for infected girdlestone procedures. Report of two cases, *J Bone Joint Surg* (1984) 66A:1466–1468

10 Collins DN, Garvin KL, Nelson CL, The use of the vastus lateralis flap in patients with intractable infection after resection arthroplasty following the use of a hip implant, *J Bone Joint Surg* (1987) 69A:510–516.

11 Little JW III, Lyons JR, the gluteus medius-tensor fascia latea flap, *Plast Recon Surg* (1983) 71:366–71.

12 May JW, Savage RC, Microvascular transfer of free tissue for closure of bone wounds of the distal lower extremity, *N Engl J Med* (1982) 306:253–257.

13 Mathes SJ, Alpert BS, Chang N, Use of the muscle flap in chronic osteomyelitis: experimental and clinical correlation, *Plast Recon Surg* (1982) 69:815–829.

14 Weiland AJ, Moore JR, Daniel RK, The efficacy of free tissue transfer in the treatment of osteomyelitis, *J Bone Joint Surg* (1984) 66A:181.

15 Gordon L, Chiu EJ, Treatment of infected non unions and segmental defects of the tibia with staged microvascular muscle transplantation and bone grafting, *J Bone Joint Surg* (1988) 70A:377–386.

16   Huntington TW, Case of bone transference, *Ann Surg* (1905) **41**:249.

17   Agiza ARH, El Kom S, Treatment of tibial osteomyelitic defects and infected pseudarthroses by the Huntington fibular transference operation, *J Bone Joint Surg* (1981) **63A**:814.

18   Gilbert A, Surgical technique vascularized transfer of the fibular shaft, *Int J Microsurg* (1979) **102**:100.

19   Moore JR, Weiland AJ, Daniel RK, Use of free vascularized bone grafts in treatment of bone tumors, *Clin Orthop Rel Res* (1983) **175**:37.

20   Taylor GI, Microvascular free bone transfer, A clinical technique, *Orthop Clin North Am* (1977) **8**:425.

21   Weiland AJ, Daniel RK, Microvascular anastomoses for bone grafts in the treatment of massive defects in bone, *J Bone Joint Surg* (1979) **61**:98–104.

22   Chacha PB, Ahmed HM, Daruwalla JS, Vascularized pedicle graft of the ipsilateral fibula for non union of the tibia with a large defect, *J Bone Joint Surg* (1981) **63B**:244–253.

23   Han CS, Wood MB, Bishop AT, et al, Vascularized bone transfer, *J Bone Joint Surg* (1992) **74A**:1441–1449.

24   Salibian AH, Anzell SH, Salyer WA, Transfer of vascularized grafts of iliac bone to the extremities, *J Bone Joint Surg* (1987) **69A**:1319–1327.

25   Jupiter JB, Bour CJ, May JW Jr, The reconstruction of defects in the femoral shaft with vascularized transfers of fibular bone, *J Bone Joint Surg* (1987) **69**:365–374.

26   Perry CR, Ellington LL, Becker A, et al, Antibiotic stability in an implantable pump, *J Orthop Res* (1986) **4**:494–498.

27   Lindsey RW, Probe R, Miclau T, et al, The effects of antibiotic-impregnated autogenic cancellous bone graft on bone healing, *Clin Orthop Rel Res* (1993) **291**:303–312.

28   Cabanela ME, Open cancellous bone grafting of infected bone defects, *Orthop Clin North Am* (1984) **15**:427.

29   Hogeman KE, Treatment of infected bone defects with cancellous bone chip grafts, *Acta Chir Scand* **98**:576–590.

30   Sudman E, Treatment of chronic osteomyelitis by free grafts of autologous bone tissue, *Acta Orthop Scand* (1979) **50**:145.

31   Green SA, Dlabal TA, The open bone graft for septic non union, *Clin Orthop Rel Res* (1983) **180**:117–124.

32   Calkins MS, Burkhalter W, Reyes F, Traumatic segmental bone defects in the upper extremity. Treatment with exposed grafts of corticocancellous iliac crest, *J Bone Joint Surg* (1987) **69A**:19–27.

33   Christian EP, Bosse MJ, Robb G, Reconstruction of large diaphyseal defects, without free fibular transfer, in grade IIIB tibial fractures, *J Bone Joint Surg* (1989) **71A**:994–1004.

34   Bosse MJ, Robb G, Techniques for the reconstruction of large traumatic bony defects with massive autogenous cancellous bone graft, *Tech Orthop* (1992) **7**:17–25.

35   Reckling FW, Waters CH III, Treatment of non unions of fractures of the tibial diaphysis by posterolateral cortical cancellous bone grafting, *J Bone Joint Surg* (1980) **62A**:936.

36   Putti V, The operative lengthening of the femur, *JAMA* (1921) **127**:934.

37   Abbott LC, The operative lengthening of the tibial and fibula, *J Bone Joint Surg* (1927) **9**:128–152.

38   Tucker HL, Kendra JC, Kinnebrew TE, Reconstruction using the method of Ilizarov as an alternative, *Orthop Clin North Am* (1990) **21**:629–637.

39   Paley D, Current techniques of limb lengthening, *J Pediatr Orthop* (1988) **8**:73–90.

40   Paley D, Catagni MA, Argnani F, et al, Ilizarov treatment of tibial non unions with bone loss, *Clin Orthop Rel Res* (1989) **241**:146–165.

41   Calhoun JH, Distraction osteogenesis with the Ilizarov technique, *Tech Orthop* (1992) **7**:27–32.

42   Dagher F, Roukoz S, Compound tibial fractures with bone loss treated by the Ilizarov technique, *J Bone Joint Surg* (1991) **73B**:316.

43   Burri C, *Post traumatic osteomyelitis* (Stuttgart: Hans Huber Bern 1975).

44   Helfet DL, Jupiter JB, Gasser S, Indirect reduction and tension band plating of tibial non union with deformity, *J Bone Joint Surg* (1992) **74A**:1286–1297.

45   Wiss D, Johnson DL, Miao M, Compression plating for nonunion after failed external fixation of open tibial fractures, *J Bone Joint Surg* (1992) **74A**:1279–1285.

46   Christiansen NO, Kuntscher intramedullary reaming and nail fixation for nonunion of fracture of the femur and the tibia, *J Bone Joint Surg* (1973) **55B**: 312–318.

47   Lottes JO, Medullary nailing of the tibia with the triflange nail, *Clin Orthop* (1974) **105**:253–266

48   Foster RJ, Dixon GL, Bach AW, et al, Internal fixation of fractures and non unions of the humeral shaft. Indications and results in a multicenter study, *J Bone Joint Surg* (1985) **67A**:857–864.

49   Galpin RD, Veith RG, Hansen ST, Treatment of failures after plating of tibial fractures, *J Bone Joint Surg* (1986) **68A**:1231–1236.

50   Fischer MD, Gustilo RB, Varecka TF, The timing of flap coverage, bone grafting, and intramedullary nailing in patients who have a fracture of the tibial shaft with extensive soft tissue injury, *J Bone Joint Surg* (1991) **73A**:1316–1322.

51   Perry CR, Rames RD, Pearson RL, Treatment of septic tibial non-unions with local antibiotics and an intramedullary nail, *Orthop Trans* (1989) **12**: 657.

52   Sledge SL, Johnson KD, Henley MB, et al, Intramedullary nailing with reaming to treat non-union of the tibia, *J Bone Joint Surg* (1989) **71A**:1004–1119.

53   Perry CR, Pearson RL, Local antibiotic delivery in the treatment of bone and joint infections, *Clin Orthop Rel Res* (1991) **263**:215–226.

7
OPERATIVE MANAGEMENT OF INFECTED JOINTS AND ARTHROPLASTIES

Infected joints and infected arthroplasties present a set of problems which differ from those encountered in the management of osteomyelitis. Unlike osteomyelitis of long bones, in which achieving stability is key, one of the goals of management of an infected joint or arthroplasty is to maintain motion. Arthrodesis is performed only as a last resort, when disabling instability is present or motion is painful. Unlike osteomyelitis of a long bone, when an infected joint or arthroplasty presents shortly after the onset of symptoms, rapid control of infection decreases functional loss. The typical patient with osteomyelitis is young, with normal host defenses. The typical patient with an infected arthroplasty is elderly, with compromised host defenses. An integral part of the management of osteomyelitis is complete débridement of necrotic bone and foreign bodies. Patients with an infected arthroplasty have a large foreign body, excision of which can result in extreme disability; therefore, we try to salvage the prosthesis when possible.

Infected joints

Management of the majority of acutely infected joints is drainage of the joint and antibiotic therapy. Chronically infected joints (ie, permanent extraarticular damage) are managed in two stages: stage 1, control of the infection; and stage 2, stabilization of the joint with arthrodesis or a total joint arthroplasty. Subacutely infected joints (ie, irreversible intraarticular damage) are managed as acutely infected joints initially. Reconstructive procedures are performed at a later date, when the extent of intraarticular damage has been determined.

Drainage of acutely infected joints in which the pathogenic organism is a Gram positive aerobe is achieved by repeated aspiration, arthroscopy, or incision and exploration. In my hands, incision and exploration achieves the most complete drainage of the joint. I utilize repeated aspiration when the patient cannot withstand a surgical procedure, and when multiple joints are involved. Although there have been no prospective randomized comparisons, the impression among orthopedic surgeons is that the results following repeated aspiration are not as good as those following incision and drainage, or arthroscopy.[1] Arthroscopic management of infected knees represents a sort of compromise between repeated aspiration, and incision and drainage.

All subacute and chronic infections, and those infections caused by anaerobes, Gram negative organisms, mycobacteria, and fungi, are managed with incision, exploration, synovectomy, and débridement.

Technique: repeated aspiration

Indications for repeated aspiration are: multiple infected joints; and a systemically ill patient who cannot withstand surgery. This method can be used only when the joints involved are easily aspirated (ie, obesity and involvement of the hip are relative contraindications) and the infection is acute and caused by Gram positive organisms, Gonococcus, or Lyme disease. A large bore needle, ie, 14–18 gauge, and 50 ml Luer lock syringe is used to aspirate the joint. It may be necessary to use more than one syringe in order to evacuate the joint entirely. When this is the case, a needle holder is used to stabilize the hub of the needle while the syringes are exchanged. It is important to note whether the material obtained from the joint flows through the needle freely. If not, and symptoms continue, assume that drainage has not been complete and an incision and exploration are necessary. After the joint has been drained, the last syringe is removed and replaced with one containing saline. The joint is injected with the saline and then aspirated.

Follow up: repeated aspiration

Follow up consists of monitoring the patient to determine whether management is effective. Swelling erythema and pain should subside. In cases in which the effusion recurs, aspiration is repeated at daily or twice daily intervals. In cases in which symptoms have not resolved within one to three days, incision and drainage are indicated. Immobilization of the joint is not necessary. Antibiotics are continued for a minimum of three weeks.

Complications: repeated aspiration

The major complication of repeated aspiration in the management of an infected joint is incomplete drainage of the joint. Incomplete drainage is due to the formation of loculations which cannot be drained with a single needle stick, or due to the intraarticular material having debris in it which impedes its flow through the needle. The most common sequela of incomplete drainage is that an acute infection becomes a subacute infection, with destruction of the intraarticular structures, in particular the articular cartilage. Eventually an inadequately drained infected joint will become chronically infected, with osteomyelitis and the destruction of surrounding ligaments and capsule. The best way to minimize the incidence of these complications is to have a low threshold for incision and exploration.

Technique: arthroscopic drainage

Although theoretically almost any joint can be drained arthroscopically, this technique is used most frequently in the management of infected knees. The arthroscope is inserted via portals on either side of the patellar tendon. The joint is examined for intraarticular pathology, in particular softening of the articular cartilage and collections of adherent fibrin debris. Following arthroscopic lavage, a pituitary rongeur is introduced through one of the portals. It is positioned in the suprapatellar pouch, where it is palpated. The pituitary rongeur is pushed through a small stab wound at its tip and its jaws are used to grasp a large drain. The drain is pulled into the joint and positioned with the rongeur. When continuous irrigation is required, an inflow tube is positioned using the same technique. At the conclusion of the procedure the portals are closed to obtain an air tight system.[2,3]

Follow up: arthroscopic drainage

Constant suction is applied to the drains, and the output is monitored. When the drain output falls to less than 10 ml per 8 hours, the drains are pulled. When continuous irrigation is used, the joint is distended with physiologic saline at a rate of 5–10 ml per hour for 4 hours. The inflow tube are then clamped and suction is applied via the outflow tube for four hours. The inflow and outflow is carefully measured. If fluid is accumulating in the joint, irrigation is stopped. In cases in which the outflow catheter is occluded, the catheter is repositioned or replaced. The inflow tubes are removed by the fourth postoperative day. The outflow catheters are left in place an additional one to four days, based on the amount of drainage.

Complications: arthroscopic drainage

Complications include occlusion of the drainage catheters, and infection of inflow tubes. Occlusion of the outflow catheters is managed by replacement or repositioning. Superinfection of catheters with resistant organisms is the major complication of inflow–outflow drainage. The incidence of superinfection is minimized by not using antibiotics in the irrigant, and by removing the catheters as soon as possible. Superinfection is indicated by cellulitis localized to the area around the catheters. When this occurs, the catheters are removed, a sample from the area

is cultured, and the appropriate antibiotic therapy is initiated. Unfortunately, the pathogenic organisms are frequently *Candida* or resistant *Pseudomonas*. After the catheters are removed, the patient is carefully monitored for any signs that the resistant organisms have seeded the joint, ie, increasing pain and effusion. When this occurs incision and drainage are performed.

Technique: incision, drainage, synovectomy, and débridement

Incision and exploration are the simplest methods is to ensure that the joint has been completely drained. The surgical approach is based on the surgeon's preference, but it must allow adequate visualization of the joint. I use an anteromedial approach for the ankle, a vertical midline skin incision, and a median parapatellar capsular incision for the knee, the Watson-Jones or Smith-Petersen approach for the hip, an anterior or Smith-Petersen approach for the sacroiliac joint, a volar "carpal tunnel" approach for the wrist, the Kocher-J approach (utilizing the interval between the brachioradialis and extensor carpi radialis longus) for the elbow, and a deltopectoral approach for the shoulder. Frequently, fibrinous material is found adhering to the articular surface; this material is débrided. The joint is carefully inspected to determine whether it has been damaged (ie, is the infection subacute)?

In cases in which the infection is subacute, chronic, or caused by anaerobes, Gram negative organisms, mycobacteria, or fungi, a synovectomy is performed. Synovium is removed with a rongeur and sharp dissection from the capsule and intraarticular structures. Flexion, extension and rotation of the joint increases the exposure, but despite our best efforts, invariably some capsular synovium is left behind. The inflamed synovium will bleed actively; therefore, perioperative blood loss must be closely monitored. In addition to the capsular synovium, there is almost always overgrowth of the cartilage with synovium. This is similar to the pannus of rheumatoid arthritis, and starts at the margins of the articular cartilage. The pannus is gently curetted from the articular surface. Under the advancing front of pannus the articular cartilage is present, but soft. Closer to the articular margin, the articular cartilage is completely absent, and subchondral bone lies under the pannus. If the infection is chronic, or caused by mycobacteria or fungi, there frequently is necrotic material and intraosseous cysts, which must be débrided.

After the joint has been drained and, if necessary, a synovectomy and débridement have been performed, it is irrigated and closed over large bore suction drains. Closure is usually in two layers. In the case of the knee, when a median parapatellar capsular approach has been used, it is important to repair the medial retinaculum, to prevent lateral subluxation of the patella.

Infection of the metacarpophalangeal joint secondary to direct inoculation is an entity which is frequently encountered, and which has two unique characteristics. (1) There is usually more than one pathogenic organism and there is a high incidence of anaerobes, specifically *Eikenella corrodens*. (2) Frequently the infection has been neglected for several days and presents as a chronic septic arthritis (ie, there is extraarticular involvement, including osteomyelitis of the metacarpal head and destruction of the collateral ligaments). The skin incision is directly midline and dorsal. The extensor expansion is divided sharply in line with the skin incision. The metacarpophalangeal joint is flexed to obtain exposure of the metacarpal head. A nick, or indentation in the articular cartilage, is specifically looked for and if found is curetted. The joint is débrided, irrigated and if the infection appears to be aggressive and advanced, packed open. In cases in which management has been initiated early, the wound is closed over a small suction drain. Care is taken to repair the extensor expansion. In cases in which there is destruction of the joint, an external fixater can be used to distract and immobilize the metacarpophalangeal joint in 30° of flexion.

Follow up: incision, drainage, synovectomy, and débridement

In the immediate perioperative period, the patient is carefully observed for signs of abscess formation. When a synovectomy is performed, the postoperative blood loss and hematocrit are closely monitored. The drains are removed when drainage decreases to less than 10 ml per 8 hours. In cases in which the infection is acute or subacute, continuous passive motion is used. When the infection is chronic or caused by mycobacteria or fungi, the joint is immobilized for one to two weeks. Early active physical therapy is important in infections of the metacarpophalangeal joint with emphasis on metacarpophalangeal flexion. Antibiotics are administered for a minimum of three weeks (often longer) in acute infections and six weeks in chronic infections. Mycobacterial and fungal infections require an extended period of antibiotic therapy.

Complications: incision, drainage, synovectomy, and débridement

Complications of incision and drainage of an infected joint include failure to cure the infection, postinfectious arthritis, instability, and a neuropathic joint. Persistent infection is indicated by swelling, effusion, continued osteolysis, and a persistently elevated erythrocyte sedimentation rate. Persistent swelling and effusion may be due to postinfectious arthritis. A persistently elevated erythrocyte sedimentation rate and osteolysis are indications of persistent infection, but infection can be present even if these findings are absent. The most accurate method of ruling out infection is aspiration or synovial biopsy of the joint. When there is persistent infection it is assumed to be chronic; ie, there is extraarticular involvement. Radiographs and either CT scans or MRI scans are obtained to rule out previously unidentified foci of infection. The joint is explored, repeat synovectomy and débridement are performed, and material obtained from the joint is cultured. Reculturing determines the presence of previously unrecognized pathogenic organisms, and whether antibiotic sensitivities have changed.

Postinfectious arthritis is managed nonoperatively with nonsteroidal antiinflammatory drugs. Frequently, symptoms will slowly diminish and eventually become tolerable. In cases in which nonoperative management is not successful, arthrodesis, excisional arthroplasty, or prosthetic arthroplasty are performed. In general, arthrodesis and excisional arthroplasty have a higher incidence of long term suppression of infection but result in greater loss of function than prosthetic arthroplasty.[4,5] Prosthetic arthroplasty is reserved for knees and hips. The painful ankle, sacroiliac joint, and wrist are managed with arthrodesis. The painful elbow and shoulder are managed with arthrodesis or excisional arthroplasty.

Instability frequently accompanies postinfectious arthritis and is managed with arthrodesis or, when the hip or knee are involved, total joint arthroplasty. A constrained knee prosthesis is used for unstable knees. The risks of arthroplasty in the management of postinfectious arthritis of the hip are illustrated by a study reported by Cherney and Amstutz.[6] In this study a series of 33 patients with a history of septic hip underwent total hip arthroplasty. Among these 33 were 9 patients with severe postinfectious arthritis following hematogenous septic arthritis. One patient had a one stage arthroplasty; the remaining eight underwent a two stage arthroplasty. Six of the nine patients had no evidence of infection following arthroplasty. Infection recurred in three patients, including the one who underwent a one stage arthroplasty. The authors conclude that "an average success rate of 70% cannot be considered perfect but, in view of the improved function that is possible, total hip-joint replacement compares very favorably with the cure rates of 80 to 90% that have been reported for infections treated by Girdlestone resection arthroplasty". They go on to point out that with

changes in their protocol (eg, adding antibiotics to the PMMA) the success rate could be increased to a level equal to that of Girdlestone resection. Kim and Kim et al reported similar results in two series of patients who underwent total hip arthroplasty for tuberculous arthritis of the hip or total knee arthroplasty for tuberculous arthritis of the knee.[7,8] In the hip series, 44 hips were implanted in 38 patients with quiescent tuberculosis. The disease was activated in six patients. All of the patients in whom the disease was activated had been actively infected in the ten years prior to total hip arthroplasty.

Neuropathic joint, or Charcot joint, is a complication of joint sepsis that occurs most frequently in diabetic patients. Although any joint can develop neuropathic changes, it is most common in the joints of the foot, the ankle, and the knee. On physical examination the joint is found to be swollen, erythematous, and warm. Pain is usually, but not always, absent. The radiographic hallmark of a neuropathic joint is exuberant bone formation combined with osteolysis. Left untreated, neuropathic changes progress to complete destruction of the joint. In many cases it is difficult to determine whether there is residual infection. When residual infection is present, the outcome is often amputation. When the diagnosis of neuropathic joint is made early, prior to loss of alignment of the joint, a total contact cast is applied and the patient is kept strictly nonweight bearing. The patient is monitored for signs of infection. If these signs occur, the cast is removed so that the extremity can be examined. At four week intervals the cast is removed. When the joint is no longer swollen and hot, the extremity is measured for a "clam shell brace" and a cast is reapplied until the brace is fabricated. If the joint is still swollen and hot the total contact cast is reapplied. Usually the time in a full contact cast is considerably longer than six months. Once the brace is applied, the weight bearing status is slowly increased. The joint is examined every several weeks; if signs of inflammation recur,

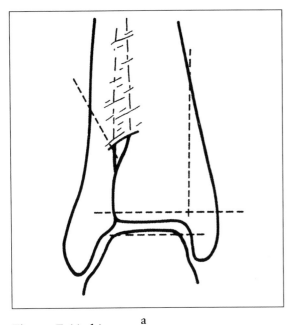 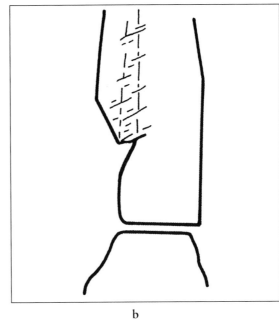

a   b

Figure 7.1(a,b)

Arthrodesis of an ankle. The fibula, medial malleolus, and articular surfaces of the talus and distal tibia are excised.

the brace is discontinued and a cast is reapplied. When all goes well the joint fuses spontaneously.

Joints which have subluxed, dislocated, or in which alignment has been lost are managed with arthrodesis. The one exception is the foot. Subluxed tarsometatarsal and midtarsal joints can frequently be managed with molded shoes after the inflammation has resolved. My experience has been that ankle arthrodesis is very acceptable to the patient. Knee arthrodesis results in significant limitation of activity (eg, the patient cannot sit in a movie theater or airplane seat, and driving an auto is difficult unless the seat is set back) and is not acceptable to the patient. Therefore, arthrodesis of the knee is performed only as a last resort. That hip arthrodesis is a good procedure is supported by a study reported by Callaghan et al.[9] In this study 28 patients who underwent hip fusion at a young age for a variety of reasons were followed for

17–50 years. The overall good results and patient acceptance indicate that hip fusion is a viable method of management of the unstable hip in the young patient. In my experience, hip arthrodesis has not been necessary because function following a Girdlestone procedure is acceptable.

Technique: arthrodesis of the ankle

External fixation is used in arthrodesis of the ankle where there is a history of infection. An external fixator has two advantages over internal fixation. It can be compressed following surgery, and no foreign material (ie, screws and plates) is left in an area in which there may be a latent infection. Through a midlateral incision, the distal 4 cm of the fibula is excised subperiosteally. Through a medial incision, the medial malleolus is excised. The articular surface of the distal tibia

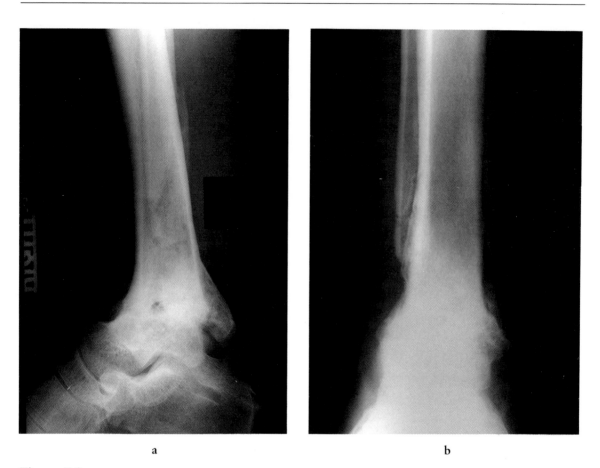

a   b

Figure 7.2

(a) Anteroposterior and (b) lateral radiographs of a fused ankle.

and talus are removed with an osteotome, creating two flat opposed cancellous surfaces (Fig. 7.1). Bone graft is not used because of the risk of activation of a latent infection. A large pin unilateral frame is applied medially. Pins are inserted in the tibia, the talus and the calcaneus. A large pin unilateral frame is used because small wire circular frames are bulkier, frequently prevent weight bearing because they extend distal to the sole of the foot, and prevent radiographic assessment of the arthrodesis site. I try to position the ankle with the tibia 0–5 mm forward on the talus, in neutral flexion, 0–5° of valgus, and 0–5° of external rotation[10] (Fig. 7.2). Initial compression with the large pin unilateral frame is achieved under direct vision. Fluoroscopy is utilized to confirm pin placement and alignment. When adequate alignment has been achieved, the medial and lateral wounds are closed over drains and a compression dressing is applied.

Follow up: arthrodesis of the ankle

The patient is instructed to keep the pin sites clean with swabs and by washing the fixator and leg with tap water. Radiographs are obtained at two week intervals in order to determine if there has been: any change in align-ment; lysis around the pins; or changes at the arthrodesis site. If it appears that there has been absorption of bone at the arthrodesis site, the fixator is used to compress the arthrodesis site at a rate of between 0.5 and 1 mm per day. When resistance is encountered with compres-sion, the rate of compression is slowed or discon-tinued. Overcompression can result in loss of alignment. When trabeculae are seen crossing the fusion site, the fusion is solid and the fixator is removed. In equivocal cases, tomograms are obtained or the fixator is dynamized. Dy-namization of a fixator denotes loosening of the fixator in such a way that alignment is main-tained, but stresses are transmitted across the arthrodesis site. If the arthrodesis is not healed there is a gradual increase in pain with activity following dynamization. After the fixator has been removed nonweight bearing is maintained for one to three weeks, and then advanced as tolerated.

Complications: arthrodesis of the ankle

The major complications of ankle arthrodesis are failure of fusion, infection, and loosening of the pins. Failure of fusion has a number of etiologies: premature removal of the frame; failure to com-press the frame; loss of alignment due to over-compression; or pin breakage and loosening of the frame. To correct any one of these, revision surgery is required (Fig. 7.3). Loosening of the pins is frequently the factor which limits the length of time that the frame remains in place. Loosening is almost always due to pin tract infec-tion and is indicated radiographically by osteo-lysis around the pins. To minimize the incidence of this complication: use good technique when inserting the pins, ie, predrill to avoid heat necro-sis of bone; relieve skin tension around the pins following closure; and insist on good postopera-tive pin care. When a pin site infection occurs, daily whirlpool and broad spectrum oral antibio-tics (eg, cefazolin) are started.

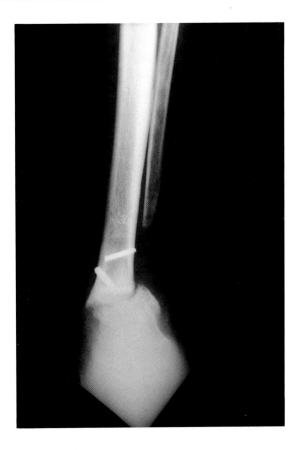

Figure 7.3

Failure of fusion. The nonunion should be taken down, the ankle realigned and a fixator reapplied. Because of a history of infection the site is not bone grafted.

Infection of the arthrodesis site often repre-sents reactivation of a latent infection. Since bone graft was not utilized and there are no fixa-tion devices in the arthrodesis site, débridement is seldom necessary. Abscesses are incised and drained, systemic antibiotics are started and the arthrodesis site is compressed. In many cases when fusion is successful the signs of infection disappear.

Technique: arthrodesis of the knee

External fixation has the same advantages in knee arthrodesis that it does in ankle arthrodesis (ie, the fixator can be compressed postoperatively, and no foreign material is left in the wound). The method of choice is a large pin unilateral frame applied to the anterior aspect of the leg. Small wire circular frames are valuable when, in addition to arthrodesis of the knee, the tibia must be lengthened, or there is angular deformity which must be corrected. The bulk of small wire circular frames necessitates wide hip abduction while weight bearing and limits the patient's mobility; therefore, their use is restricted to selected cases (eg, when there is angular deformity which must be corrected with the frame). In my experience, arthrodesis of a knee with latent osteomyelitis by means of an intramedullary nail is associated with a high incidence of activation of latent osteomyelitis and fracture of the tibia at the distal tip of the nail; therefore, I no longer perform this procedure.

The distal surface of the femur and proximal surface of the tibia are exposed through a medial, lateral, or anterior incision. Usually there have been prior surgeries which dictate the surgical approach. The articular surfaces of the distal femur and proximal tibia are excised with an oscillating saw, leaving two flat apposable surfaces. The patella may be left *in situ* or used as a source of bone graft. Bone graft is not used if there are any signs of active infection. The ideal position for fusion is 10° of flexion and 5° of valgus. The fixator is applied with a minimum of three pins in the tibia and femur. After the fixator has been applied it is used to compress the arthrodesis site under direct vision (Fig. 7.4). When satisfactory alignment and compression of the arthrodesis site have been achieved, the wound is closed over suction drains.

Follow up: arthrodesis of the knee

As in ankle arthrodesis, pin care is crucial. Radiographs are obtained every two weeks: to assess alignment; to determine if osteolysis has occurred around the pins; and to document the presence of consolidation at the arthrodesis site. One to two weeks after surgery the arthrodesis site is compressed 0.5–1 mm a day until resistance is met. When resistance is met the rate of compression is slowed or discontinued. Successful fusion is indicated radiographically by trabeculae crossing the arthrodesis site. In equivocal cases, tomograms of the fusion are obtained. Following fixator removal, nonweight bearing is maintained for two weeks; weight bearing is then increased as tolerated.

Complications: arthrodesis of the knee

The major complications of arthrodesis of the knee are identical to those of arthrodesis of the ankle (ie, failure of fusion; infection; and loosening of the pins) and are managed in the same way.

Infected arthroplasties

Management of an infected arthroplasty is via one of four basic techniques: long term suppression of infection with systemic antibiotics; salvage of the prosthesis with minimal débridement and administration of antibiotics; excisional arthroplasty or fusion; and one or two stage revision.

Long term suppression

Long term suppression of infection in the management of infected arthroplasties is reserved for a specific group of patients. The pathogenic organism must be sensitive to antibiotics which can be administered orally and which the patient tolerates. The joint must be asymptomatic, this usually means that the patient has low demands. There must not be chronic drainage, as this may become superinfected with resistant organisms in the presence of extended antibiotic administra-

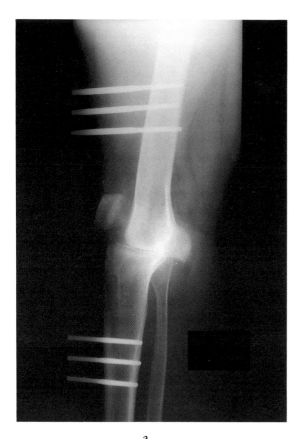 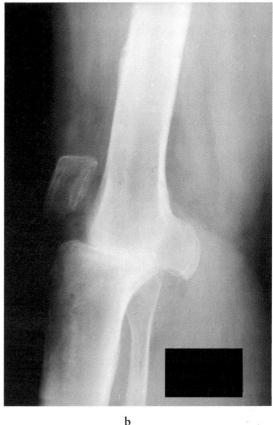

a   b

Figure 7.4(a,b)

Lateral radiographs of a knee. The joint surfaces have been excised, and a large pin unilateral external fixator has been used to compress the arthrodesis site.

tion. The patient must understand that lysis around the prosthesis may compromise the result of a revision if it becomes necessary.

Salvage of the prosthesis

The theoretical advantage of salvaging an infected arthroplasty is that in some cases it will last longer and function better than a revision arthroplasty. Unfortunately, the rate of success has been very low. The futility of systemic antibiotic administration and leaving the pros-

thesis in situ is illustrated by several series. Walker and Schurman reported 14 patients with total knee arthroplasty infections managed with limited débridement and antibiotic administration.[11] In two of four patients with perioperative infections long term suppression was achieved. Treatment failed in all the patients with infections occurring after the perioperative period. The authors conclude that "this method is applicable only in cases of immediate postoperative infection and uniformly unsuccessful in infections occurring beyond the perioperative period". Schoifet and Morrey reported a series of 27 patients with 31 infected total knee arthroplasties managed with limited débridement (the components were left in situ) and systemic antibiotic therapy.[12] Infection recurred in 24 or 77% of the knees. They correlated poor prognosis with: increased duration of infection; Gram negative organisms; and a hinged prosthesis. Grogan et al reported 13 patients with infected total knee arthroplasties.[13] Twelve patients were managed initially with antibiotics and limited débridement. The prosthesis was salvaged in only four cases. Similar rates of success have been reported by other authors.[14,15] Wilson et al reported the highest rate of success using limited débridement and systemic antibiotic administration.[16] In their series of 31 infected total knee arthroplasties, limited débridement consisted of repeated aspiration in 8 knees and arthrotomy in 23 knees. Antibiotics were administered intravenously. Infection was suppressed in 17 patients. Unlike other authors, Wilson et al found no correlation between the incidence of suppression and the length of time from the index surgery and the onset of symptoms of infection. They found that the pathogenic organism did correlate with the prognosis. Most significantly, their management was successful in all five patients infected with Streptococcus.

I reported a series of 12 patients with infected knee or hip arthroplasties managed with débridement, retention of the prosthesis, and local antibiotic administration via an implantable pump.[17] Follow up was for a minimum of three years, and suppression of infection was achieved in 10 of the 12 patients. This series has since expanded to 43 patients.[18] Thirty-one patients had knee arthroplasties. Twelve patients had hip arthroplasties. All 43 patients had positive cultures obtained either from wound drainage or from an aspirate. Pathogenic organisms were: Staphylococcus aureus in 15 cases; Staphylococcus epidermidis in 13 cases; Gram negative organisms in four cases; Staphylococcus aureus or Staphylococcus epidermidis with a Gram negative organism in six cases; and Enterococcus in five cases. Ten patients were immunocompromised, four were diabetics, five

were on steroids for autoimmune diseases, and one patient had biliary cirrhosis. Two patients died from unrelated medical problems, leaving 41 patients. Follow up ranges from 5 to 53 months.

Suppression of infection was defined purely on a clinical basis. All 41 patients had presented with an obviously infected prosthesis, as evidenced by pain, swelling, erythema and drainage. A result was considered successful if: there were no signs of infection after antibiotics had been discontinued; the joint had a painless range of motion; and the patient could bear full weight without discomfort. Based on these parameters there were eight failures. The identity of the organism correlated with failure of therapy. Methicillin resistant Staphylococcus aureus or epidermidis was the pathogen in three of the eight patients in whom therapy failed. Gram negative pathogens did not adversely affect the prognosis. Immunosuppression did not affect the final result in that only two of the failures were immunocompromised.

Two of the eight failures of therapy were treated as chronic infections (ie, the pump was left in place, the joint was resected, and a revision arthroplasty was performed as a second stage). Both are doing well. Two of the eight failures of therapy were treated with arthrodesis. Two were treated with resection of the prosthesis without arthrodesis or reinsertion of a prosthesis. Two are being managed by long term suppression with oral antibiotics. The complication unique to local antibiotic therapy with an implantable pump is infection of the pump site or delivery catheters. Four of the 41 patients developed this complication.

Technique: salvage of the prosthesis with débridement and local administration of antibiotics

In cases in which there are no indications of involvement of the bone–prosthesis interface, we attempt to salvage the prosthesis with débridement and local antibiotic administration via an implantable pump. The prosthesis is left in situ when the following conditions are met: the prosthesis is in good position; the duration of infection is less than six weeks; and there are no radiographic signs of periprosthetic lysis. The pump is implanted in the ipsilateral lower quadrant of the abdomen when the knee is involved, and in the contralateral quadrant when the hip is involved. The joint is exposed and débrided via the incision through which the prosthesis was inserted. Necrotic tissue is removed, but a complete synovectomy is not necessary. The interface between the bone and the femoral and tibial components is exposed and examined to determine definitively whether the prosthesis is loose. If it is loose, the prosthesis cannot be salvaged and it is excised and replaced with a PMMA–antibiotic spacer. The outflow catheters are tunneled subcutaneously and brought through the joint capsule, where they are held in place with fine absorbable suture. Closure is accomplished over large suction drains. When closing the knee it is necessary to repair the medial retinaculum to prevent postoperative subluxation of the patella.

Follow-up: salvage of the prosthesis with débridement and local administration of antibiotics

Systemic antibiotics are continued while the patient is in the hospital. Continuous passive motion is utilized for the first two postoperative days to prevent loculations from forming. The drains are left in place until drainage is less than 10 ml per 8 hours. Drainage at a rate greater than 10 ml per 8 hours more than five days after pump implantation is an indicator that there is persistent infection. Once the drains have been removed, the patient is followed closely for reaccumulation of fluid in the joint. Reaccumulation of a joint effusion, increasing pain, and an erythrocyte sedimentation rate which remains elevated indicate persistent infection. If swelling and pain gradually subside, and the erythrocyte

sedimentation rate falls, the pump is allowed to run dry after eight to ten weeks. If the patient remains asymptomatic after two to four weeks with no local antibiotics having been delivered to the joint, the pump can be removed as an outpatient procedure.

Complications: salvage of the prosthesis with débridement and local administration of antibiotics

Complications include failure to suppress the infection and pump site infection. Failure to suppress the infection is managed by two stage revision of the joint. The pump is left in situ. The prosthesis is removed and the joint débrided. A PMMA–antibiotic spacer and the outflow catheters of the pump are left in the joint. A revision is performed if the infection is successfully suppressed. Pump site infection is managed with aspiration of the pocket and oral antibiotics. In some cases it is necessary to remove the pump.

Excisional arthroplasty or arthrodesis

Excisional arthroplasty or arthrodesis results in a significant loss of function, and therefore is performed only as a final resort in the management of infected total joints. The concept is that the removal of implants and cement maximizes the effectiveness of host defenses, increasing the chance of long term suppression of infection. The trade off is shortening, in all cases, and a flail joint when arthrodesis is not performed.

Excisional arthroplasty is considered primarily in the management of infected elbow, shoulder, and hip prostheses. Infected ankle and knee prostheses are usually managed with arthrodesis. An additional relative indication for excisional arthroplasty verses arthrodesis is a patient with low demands. Wolfe et al reported a series of 12 patients with infected total elbow arthroplasties.[15] In nine cases the joint was resected after an unsuccessful attempt to salvage it with débridement and systemic antibiotic therapy. These results indicate that there is a low probability of successful salvage of the prosthesis, and that because resection arthroplasty is inevitable it is in the patient's best interest to do it early. In Wolfe et al's study, seven of the nine patients who had undergone resection were left with an excisional arthroplasty. Two patients underwent arthrodesis in a second procedure. The three patients whose prosthesis was not excised were maintained on suppressive oral antibiotic therapy.

Morrey and Bryan published two reports which apply to the management of the patient with infected elbow arthroplasties.[19,20] The majority of the patients in both of these reports had rheumatoid arthritis, and therefore presumably had a low level of physical demands. The first report included 33 patients undergoing revision elbow arthroplasty. Among these were three who developed an infection, and were managed with resection arthroplasty. The final result was rated as fair in all three. The second paper focused primarily on the high incidence of postoperative infection following total elbow arthroplasty. In this paper Morrey and Bryan reported 14 patients with infected elbow arthroplasties. Similar to Wolfe et al's series, when the prosthesis was left in situ, débridement and antibiotic administration successfully salvaged the prosthesis in only one case. Two patients were managed successfully with débridement, systemic antibiotics and revision arthroplasty as a second stage. The remaining 11 patients were left with resection arthroplasty and ultimately had an acceptable result. These three studies indicate that resection elbow arthroplasty is well tolerated.

Most of the experience with excisional arthroplasty of the shoulder has been with tumors of the proximal humerus and scapula.[21,22] Resection of the proximal humerus and glenoid is occasionally necessary in the management of infected shoulder arthroplasties. In my experience fusion of the shoulder is seldom necessary, and results in unacceptable shortening.

The hip is seldom fused following excision of an infected prosthesis. In many cases there has been significant loss of bone and fusion will result in unacceptable shortening. In addition, arthrodesis of the hip is a difficult procedure with significant risk for the patient. Excisional arthroplasty of the hip, or the Girdlestone procedure, has a long history. It was first described by White in 1849 as a treatment for a septic hip. In 1928 Girdlestone described excisional arthroplasty in the management of tuberculous arthritis of the hip.[23] The procedure is still performed according to his technique whenever possible. Grauer et al reported a series of 43 patients with resection arthroplasties of the hip.[5] Thirty-three of the resection arthroplasties were performed for septic hip arthroplasties. The procedure was successful in suppressing infection in all but three cases. However, there was significant shortening in all cases, and all of the patients had to use a cane, crutches, or a walker for ambulation. Grauer et al concluded that there was a direct correlation between the patient's postoperative activity and the amount of femur salvaged. Canner et al reported a series of 52 infected total hip arthroplasties.[14] Thirty-three patients were managed with excisional arthroplasty. The infection was suppressed in 27 of these 33 patients, but the clinical result was rated as satisfactory in only 20.

Arthrodesis is used more frequently than excisional arthroplasty to manage infected total knee arthroplasties. However, in sedentary patients arthrodesis not only is not necessary but also makes it difficult to position the patient in a wheelchair. Falahee et al reported a series of 26 patients with infected total knee arthroplasties who were managed with excisional arthroplasty.[24] Following resection the extremity was immobilized in a long leg cast for an average of 5.5 months. Two knees spontaneously ankylosed. Fifteen of the 24 patients who were ambulatory prior to resection arthroplasty were able to walk following surgery; however, the majority used a brace. The authors conclude that resection arthroplasty "can provide a very comfortable useful range of motion of the knee for the disabled sedentary patient", but that it is "least suitable for patients who have had relatively minor disability before the total joint replacement".

Technique: excisional arthroplasty of the elbow, shoulder, hip, and knee

The key to suppression of infection following excisional arthroplasty is complete removal of all necrotic bone and cement, dead space management, and appropriate antibiotic administration. The surgical approach is the same as that used when the prosthesis was implanted. A variety of osteotomes (straight, curved and flexible), curette (straight, curved and reverse), cement extraction hooks, a fiberoptic light (for visualization of the medullary canal), and a high speed burr facilitate removal of the prosthesis and the cement. Fluoroscopy is useful to identify intramedullary fragments of cement. Frequently the prosthesis is loose, but abundant scar tissue and fibrosis of the joint capsule prevent subluxation of the joint and extraction of the components.[25] Excision of this scar tissue and capsule may be necessary in order to extract the components. When the prosthesis is not loose, osteotomizing the femur, in order to remove the femoral stem of a total hip arthroplasty, or the tibia, in order to remove the tibial component of a total knee arthroplasty, may be the least destructive way of removing the prosthesis. To osteotomize the femur, drill holes are placed at regular intervals in the anterolateral cortex extending to at least 5 cm distal to the tip of the prosthesis or cement restricter. These holes are connected with a sagittal saw. A broad osteotome is placed in the osteotomy and used to gently lever open the osteotomy site, freeing the prosthesis, and allowing its removal. This often results in a minimally displaced fracture which extends distally. Once the prosthesis is removed the osteotomy reduces spontaneously, and is stabilized with a cerclage wire. To osteotomize the tibia, the identical procedure is performed on the anteromedial cortex

of the tibia. As in the femur, the holes are connected with a sagittal saw, and the osteotomy is levered open. Complete removal of the cement is confirmed radiographically.

When the prosthesis has been removed, samples of material obtained from the bone–prosthesis interface are sent for culture. I routinely send specimens for aerobic, anaerobic, fungal and acid fast culture. It is important that antibiotics are not administered prior to obtaining material for culture.

Dead space is filled with PMMA-antibiotic beads. The cavity is packed loosely, so that surrounding soft tissue can contract postoperatively. The wound is closed over two large bore drains. If the hip is involved a distal femoral traction pin is inserted. If the elbow or knee is involved, a compression dressing which incorporates splints is applied. The elbow is immobilized at 90°, the knee in full extension. If the involved joint is a shoulder, a shoulder immobilizer is applied.

Follow-up: excisional arthroplasty of the elbow, shoulder, hip, and knee

Bleeding from the debrided bone ends may continue for several days; therefore, the hematocrit must be carefully monitored. Antibiotics are administered a total of six weeks; they are altered according to the intraoperative cultures. The drains are left in until drainage has decreased to less than 10 ml per 8 hours, or a minimum of two weeks. At three to six weeks, beads and spacers are removed as atraumatically as possible via a small incision. The incision is closed over a drain. Ideally, the dead space has contracted to the point where new beads are not required. In cases in which beads are reinserted, they are removed after an additional three to six weeks.

If the involved joint is a hip, skeletal traction is maintained for approximately three weeks. Two to three days after surgery the patient is taken out of traction and sat up in a chair for an hour a day. Gait training is initiated when the patient is strong enough to benefit from therapy.

Radiographs in traction confirm that the hip is pulled out to length. At three weeks, skeletal traction is discontinued, and the patient sleeps in 1–2 kg of Buck's traction. If the involved joint is a knee, gait training with weight bearing as tolerated is initiated in a knee immobilizer. In the vast majority of cases it is not until two to three months after surgery that the patient begins to put significant pressure on the involved leg. Around six months a knee–ankle–foot orthosis with drop lock hinges and an appropriate size shoe lift is prescribed. If the involved joint is an elbow, a removable plastic molded splint is prescribed at one week. A hinged brace is prescribed when swelling and pain have diminished, usually around two months after surgery. If the involved joint is a shoulder, the shoulder immobilizer is continued for comfort; usually by three weeks it is no longer required, and a sling can be substituted for it. By two months no immobilization is required. Pendulum exercises are started when the patient can tolerate them, usually around one week.

Complications: excisional arthroplasty of the elbow, shoulder, hip, and knee

The two complications of excisional arthroplasty are persistent infection, and severe displacement of the resected bone ends. Persistent infection is managed with redébridement, repeat cultures, and four to six weeks of antibiotic administration. Severe displacement of the resected bone ends may result in unacceptable instability. In the upper extremity, instability may result in neurologic compromise; in the lower extremity, it may make weight bearing impossible. Instability of the upper extremity is initially managed with a sling. The shoulder may have to be supported indefinitely with a sling; the elbow often eventually can be braced. Instability of a resected hip results in unacceptable shortening of the extremity with weight bearing, the only options are to decrease weight bearing and increase the size of the shoe lift. Management

of an unstable resected knee is casting or bracing of the extremity with the bone ends in a reduced position.

Arthrodesis

Arthrodesis results in a stable joint at the expense of mobility. In the ankle, mobility is not nearly as important as it is in the knee. While I have found arthrodesis of the ankle to be very well tolerated by patients, I have found that knee arthrodesis is not. My primary indication for knee arthrodesis is a patient with an excisional arthroplasty who has pain or cannot tolerate the inherent lack of stability of a flail knee.

Rand and Bryan described arthrodesis in the management of failed total knee arthroplasty in 28 patients (25 due to infection).[26] An external fixator was used in all cases. In 20 cases the initial procedure was successful in achieving fusion. The only complication related directly to the fixator was a fracture and subsequent nonunion through a pin hole.

Puranen et al reported a series of 33 patients who underwent knee fusion with an intramedullary nail.[27] Eight patients in this series had an infected total knee arthroplasty. The authors used an open technique (ie, the knee was opened, and the femur and tibia were reamed from the knee). In the eight infected cases, the knee was débrided and the nail inserted at the same surgery; antibiotics were administered postoperatively for an average of 25 days. The authors reported that: 29 of the 33 knees in their series went on to fusion; the nail broke in the four cases in which fusion did not occur; there were no new infections; and active drainage stopped in three of the eight infected knees. They emphasize that good bone to bone contact must be obtained at the knee and that fusion with an intramedullary nail is a relatively safe procedure.

Donley et al reported a series of 21 patients who underwent arthrodesis of the knee with an intramedullary rod.[28] Among these 21 patients were 8 with an infected total knee arthroplasty.

As in the technique described by Puranen et al, the nail was inserted through the knee. However, unlike Puranen et al's technique, arthrodesis of infected knees was performed in two stages: first, débridement and administration of antibiotics; second, arthrodesis. The difficulty of knee arthrodesis with an intramedullary nail is indicated by an average operative time of 3.7 hours, and an average blood loss of 1500 ml. Donley et al's two stage technique was successful in achieving fusion and suppression of infection in seven of the eight patients who had an infected total knee arthroplasty. This higher incidence of suppression of infection argues strongly for a two stage procedure when arthrodesing an infected total knee arthroplasty with an intramedullary nail.

The seriousness of ankle arthrodesis is indicated by a paper whose primary purpose was to report a posterior approach to the ankle. In this paper, Russotti et al reported a series of 28 patients who underwent ankle arthrodesis.[29] Among them were five patients with infected total ankle arthroplasties. Bone loss from the talus precluded a tibiotalar fusion in these five patients, and they were managed with tibiocalcaneal arthrodesis. Two of these five ultimately underwent below knee amputation for uncontrollable infection and peripheral vascular disease.

The technique, follow up, and complications of arthrodesis of the knee and ankle is described above and is identical to that used for infected total joint arthroplasties. There will be more shortening with following arthrodesis for an infected total joint arthroplasty than for post-infectious arthritis. This shortening must be acceptable to the patient.

One or two stage exchange arthroplasty

Exchange arthroplasty is performed as a one or two stage procedure. In a one stage procedure, the infected prosthesis is excised, the joint débrided, and another prosthesis implanted, usually held in place with PMMA–antibiotic composite. In a two stage procedure, the infected prosthesis is excised and the joint débrided in one surgery. A prosthesis is reimplanted in a second surgery. The advantages of a one stage procedure are that morbidity due to a second procedure is minimized, and the patient does not have a flail extremity in the period of time between the débridement and revision surgeries. The disadvantages of a one stage procedure are that the rate of recurrence of infection is higher than with a two stage procedure, and that a more extensive débridement of bone and soft tissue must be performed, making reconstruction more difficult.

Buchholz et al reported the largest series of infected total joint arthroplasties (825 infected total hip arthroplasties) managed with a one stage revision.[30] Massive débridement and the use of PMMA–antibiotic composites were the key to Buchholz's technique. A variety of antibiotics were used in the composite; however, gentamicin was used most frequently. With a minimum five year follow up, Buchholz et al reported a 77% incidence of suppression of infection. These impressive results are tempered by the fact that pathogenic organisms were not isolated for 152 patients (17%), leading to the suspicion that some revisions may have been performed for aseptic loosening. Among the cases in which pathogens were isolated, the authors found that infections caused by *Pseudomonas* had an extremely poor prognosis.

In North America two stage revisions are performed more commonly than one stage revision. The hypothesis that the longer the period of time between the débridement and the revision surgery, the lower the incidence of recurrence of infection, is supported by several studies. Rand et al retrospectively reviewed 14 patients who underwent exchange arthroplasty for an infected total knee.[31] Revision was performed within two weeks of the initial debridement. Treatment was successful in suppressing infection in only 8 of the 14 patients. McDonald et al reported a series of 81 patients with septic hip arthroplasties who underwent two stage revision.[32]

PMMA–antibiotic composites were not used in the revision surgery. Infection recurred in 11 hips. The authors correlated recurrent infection with reimplantation within one year of the débridement. In addition to the length of time between débridement and the revision, retained cement and systemic antibiotic administration for less than 28 days correlated with an unsuccessful outcome. When antibiotics are delivered locally via an implantable pump, the period of time between the débridement and revision can safely be shortened. We have treated 15 patients with chronically infected total joint arthroplasties using local antibiotics delivered with an implantable pump. Six were total hip replacements. Nine were total knee replacements. All had radiographic signs of periprosthetic osteolysis and positive cultures of the joint aspirate or drainage. The infecting organisms were: *Staphylococcus aureus* or *Staphylococcus epidermidis* alone in seven cases; *Staphylococcus aureus* or *Staphylococcus epidermidis* with Gram negative organisms in three cases; and Gram negative organisms alone in five cases. Five patients were immunocompromised secondary to rheumatoid arthritis, steroids, diabetes or immunosuppression for a liver transplant. Twelve patients were treated with two stage revisions. The interval between the initial débridement and reimplantation ranged from three to five weeks. Follow up ranges from 18 to 62 months. In 12 of the 15 patients the infection has been successfully suppressed.

The highest incidence of suppression of infection achieved with two stage revisions of infected prostheses was reported by Windsor et al.[33] Their report is a follow up of a paper published by Insall et al, and includes 38 patients with infected total knee arthroplasties.[34] Systemic antibiotics were administered for a minimum of six weeks following the débridement, and the revision prosthesis was implanted an average of 55 days following débridement. Follow up ranged from 2.5 to 10 years. Four patients developed an infection after reimplantation, but only one of these was with the original organism.

These excellent results are tempered by the fact that this is a selected series; the authors carefully document 13 patients who were excluded from the study for a variety of reasons including: fulminant infection; inadequate viability of skin; and neutropenia. Clearly, the authors do not expect that two stage revision will be successful in all patients.

Technique: two stage exchange arthroplasty

The goal of the débridement surgery is to remove the prosthesis, necrotic bone, and all of the cement, while at the same time minimizing damage to viable bone and soft tissue. The technique of débridement has been described previously, under "Excisional arthroplasty or arthrodesis". When the joint is completely débrided, the dead space is filled with a PMMA–antibiotic spacer. If the involved joint is the hip, PMMA–antibiotic beads are used. If the involved joint is the knee, a PMMA–antibiotic block is placed between the tibia and femur, and remaining dead space is filled with beads. The PMMA–antibiotic spacer delivers antibiotics locally and maintains the length of surrounding soft tissue, making reimplantation of a prosthesis easier. In addition, the PMMA–antibiotic spacer, or block, in the knee often will stabilize the joint in extension, increasing the patient's mobility while he or she is waiting for the revision surgery. The block is fashioned on the back table. It is made to approximate the size and shape of the tibial component. The addition of a "stem" which projects down the medullary canal of the tibia decreases the incidence of dislocation of the block from between the tibia and femur (Figs 7.5, 7.6). If a pump has been implanted to deliver antibiotics locally, the outflow catheters are sutured in place. The wound is closed over large suction drains. If the involved joint is a hip, a distal femoral traction pin is inserted and the extremity is placed in traction.

Follow-up: one or two stage exchange arthroplasty

The surfaces of the bone bleed freely for several days; therefore, the patient's hematocrit is followed closely in the perioperative period. If antibiotics are being administered locally via a pump, systemic antibiotics are continued until the signs of cellulitis have resolved. The drains are left in place until their output falls to less than 10 ml per 8 hours. If the drainage does not decrease, the drains are removed two to three weeks after the débridement. Patients with involvement of the knee are weight bearing as tolerated in a knee immobilizer. In the majority of cases weight bearing is held to a minimum because it is not comfortable. Patients with involvement of the hip are in skeletal traction for the first week; two to three days following surgery they are taken out of traction to sit at the side of the bed for short periods of time. In the second and third week they are taken out of traction for eight hours a day to sit in a chair and stand between parallel bars. At the end of the third week the traction pin is removed; the patient sleeps with 1–2 kg of Buck's traction applied to the extremity. Weight bearing is usually minimal in the first month, as it is not comfortable.

Timing of revision surgery becomes an important issue. Factors which mitigate for early

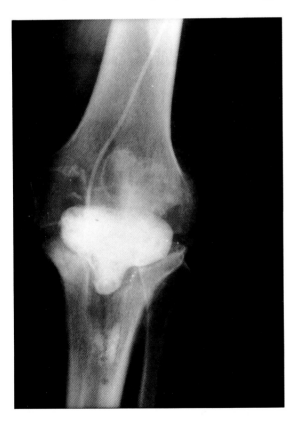

Figure 7.5

Radiograph of a débrided knee with a stemmed spacer. The stem prevents dislocation of the spacer. An outflow catheter of a pump is seen overlying the femur.

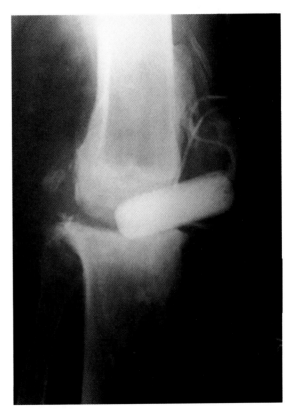

Figure 7.6

Dislocation of a PMMA–antibiotic spacer without a stem from between the femur and tibia

revision surgery are: an uncomplicated clinical course (ie, rapid resolution of cellulitis and rapid decrease in drainage); a sensitive pathogenic organism; a steadily falling erythrocyte sedimentation rate; and patient intolerance of the limited activity level due to the flail joint. If antibiotics have been administered locally via an implantable pump, revision surgery is performed as early as four weeks. The pump is left in situ, with the outflow catheters in the joint. PMMA–antibiotic composite is used as cement in the revision, and following surgery the pump is refilled for a minimum of three weeks. If antibiotics are administered systemically, revision is performed at a minimum of three months following the débridement, and again PMMA–antibiotic composite is used as cement in the revision.

Complications: one or two stage revision arthroplasty

The major complication of one or two stage revision arthroplasty is inability to eradicate the infection or recurrent infection. Some patients undergoing two stage revision arthroplasty will continue to drain and have signs of cellulitis after removal of the prosthesis, despite the fact that they are receiving antibiotics. When this happens there are two choices: (1) go back in and redébride, making sure that no cement or necrotic bone has been left behind, reculturing the wound, and implanting new spacers; (2) remove the spacers and close the wound over suction drains with the understanding that revision is no longer an option. When infection recurs after the revision, the options are to suppress the infection with oral antibiotics, or to redébride the joint and perform a second delayed revision, arthrodese the joint, or leave it flail.

References

1   Leslie BM, Harris JM, Driscoll D, Septic arthritis of the shoulder in adults, *J Bone Joint Surg* (1989) **71A**:1516–1522.

2   Gainor BJ, Instillation of continuous tube irrigation in the septic knee at arthroscopy – a technique, *Clin Orthop Rel Res* (1984) **183**:96–98.

3   Jarrett MP, Grossman L, Sadler AH, et al, The role of arthroscopy in the treatment of septic arthritis, *Arthritis Rheum* (1981) **24**:737.

4   Ahlgren SA, Gudmundsson G, Bartholdsson E, Function after removal of a septic total hip prosthesis. A survey of 27 Girdlestone hips, *Acta Orthop Scand* (1980) **51**:541–545.

5   Grauer JD, Amstutz HC, O'Carroll PF, et al, Resection arthroplasty of the hip, *J Bone Joint Surg* (1989) **71A**:669–678.

6   Cherney DL, Amstutz HC, Total hip replacement in the previously septic hip, *J Bone Joint Surg* (1983) **65A**:1256–1265.

7   Kim YH, Total knee arthroplasty for tuberculous arthritis, *J Bone Joint Surg* (1988) **70A**:1322–1330.

8   Kim YH, Han DY, Park BM, Total hip arthroplasty for tuberculous coxarthrosis, *J Bone Joint Surg* (1987) **69A**: 718–727.

9   Callaghan JJ, Brand RA, Pedersen DR, Hip arthrodesis. A long-term follow-up, *J Bone Joint Surg* (1985) **67A**:1328– 1335.

10   Buck P, Morrey BF, Chao EY, The optimum position of arthrodesis of the ankle. A gait study of the knee and ankle, *J Bone Joint Surg* (1987) **69A**:1052–1062.

11   Walker RH, Schurman DJ, Management of infected total knee arthroplasties, *Clin Orthop Rel Res* (1984) **186**:81–89.

12   Shoifet SD, Morrey BF, Treatment of infection after total knee arthroplasty by debridement with retention of the components, *J Bone Joint Surg* (1990) **72**:1383–1390.

13   Grogan TJ, Dorey F, Rollins J, et al, Deep sepsis following total knee arthroplasty. Ten-year experience at the University of California at Los Angeles medical center, *J Bone Joint Surg* (1986) **68A**:226–234.

14   Canner GC, Steinberg ME, Heppenstall RB, et al, The infected hip after total hip arthroplasty, *J Bone Joint Surg* (1984) **66A**:1393–1399.

15   Wolfe SW, Figgie MP, Inglis AE, et al, Management of infection about total elbow prostheses, *J Bone Joint Surg* (1990) **72A**:198–212.

16   Wilson MG, Kelley K, Thornhill TS, Infection as a complication of total knee replacement arthroplasty. Risk factors and treatment in sixty-seven cases, *J Bone Joint Surg* (1990) **72A**:878–883.

17   Perry CR, Pearson RL, Local antibiotics delivery in the treatment of bone and joint infections, *Clin Orthop Rel Res* (1991) **263**:213–226.

18   Perry CR, Hulsey RE, Mann FA, et al, Treatment of acutely infected arthroplasties with incision, drainage, and local antibiotics delivered via an implantable pump, *Clin Orthop Rel Res* (1992) **281**:216–223.

19   Morrey BF, Bryan RS, Infection after total elbow arthroplasty, *J Bone Joint Surg* (1983) **65A**:330–338.

20   Morrey BF, Bryan RS, Revision total elbow arthroplasty, *J Bone Joint Surg* (1987) **69A**:523–532.

21   Janecki CJ, Nelson CL, En bloc resection of the shoulder girdle: technique and indications: report of a case, *J Bone Joint Surg* (1972) **54A**:1754–1756.

22   Linberg BE, Interscapulo-thoracic resection for malignant tumors of the shoulder joint region, *J Bone Joint Surg* (1928) **10**:344–347.

23   Girdlestone GR, Acute pyogenic arthritis of the hip – an operation giving free access and effective drainage, *Lancet* (1943) 419–420.

24   Falahee MH, Mathews LS, Kaufer H, Resection arthroplasty as a salvage procedure for a knee with infection after a total arthroplasty, *J Bone Joint Surg* (1987) **69A**:1013–1020.

25   Mallory TH, Excision arthroplasty with delayed wound closure for the infected total hip replacement, *Clin Orthop* (1978) **137**:106–111.

26   Rand JA, Bryan RS, Reimplantation for the salvage of an infected total knee arthroplasty, *J Bone Joint Surg* (1983) **65A**:1081–1086.

27   Puranen J, Kortelainen P, Jalovaara P, Arthrodesis of the knee with intramedullary nail fixation, *J Bone Joint Surg* (1990) **72A**:433–442.

28   Donley BG, Mathews LS, Kaufer H, Arthrodesis of the knee with an intramedullary nail, *J Bone Joint Surg* (1991) **73A**:907–913.

29   Russotti GM, Johnson KA, Cass JR, Tibiocalcaneal arthrodesis for arthritis and deformity of the hind part of the foot, *J Bone Joint Surg* (1988) **70A**:1304–1307.

30   Buchholz HW, Elson RA, Heinert K, Antibiotic-loaded acrylic cement: current concepts, *Clin Orthop Rel Res* (1984) **190**:96–108.

31   Rand JA, Bryan RS, Chao EYS, Failed total knee arthroplasty treated by arthrodesis of the knee using the Ace Fisher apparatus, *J Bone Joint Surg* (1987) **69A**:39–45.

32   McDonald DJ, Fitzgerald RH, Ilstrup DM, Two-stage reconstruction of a total hip

arthroplasty because of infection, *J Bone Joint Surg* (1989) **71A:**823–834.

33   Windsor RE, Insall JN, Urs WK, et al, Two stage reimplantation for the salvage of total knee arthroplasty complicated by infection. Further follow-up and refinement of

indications, *J Bone Joint Surg* (1990) **72A:**272–278.

34   Insall JN, Thompson FM, Brause BD, Two stage reimplantation for the salvage of infected total knee arthroplasty, *J Bone Joint Surg* (1983) **65A:**1087–1098.

8
SPECIFIC CLINICAL PROBLEMS

The successful management of bone and joint infections requires a degree of flexibility on the part of the orthopedic surgeon. Individual medical and surgical techniques described in Chapters 4, 5, 6 and 7 are utilized, but the ideal selection and timing of each technique are not always obvious. This chapter outlines the way that I approach specific clinical problems. The clinical problems are: focal osteomyelitis with bony continuity; infected fractures; infected nonunion of long bones; infected segmental defects of long bones; nonunion with latent osteomyelitis; lower extremity infection in the diabetic patient; acute septic arthritis; chronic septic arthritis; infection in association with a hemoglobinopathy; and infected arthroplasty.

Management consists of: débridement; soft tissue coverage; dead space management; and antibiotic administration. Stabilization is obviously not necessary, as the bone is in continuity. Management is staged. Stage I – necrotic tissue and implants are débrided, dead space is temporarily obliterated with PMMA–antibiotic beads, and antibiotic administration (either systemic or local via a pump) is initiated. Soft tissue coverage is usually achieved with primary closure; occasionally free or local tissue transfers are necessary. Stage II – the beads are removed and autogenous cancellous graft into which antibiotics have been mixed is used to obliterate the dead space; antibiotics are continued for an additional three weeks.

Focal osteomyelitis with the bone in continuity

Focal osteomyelitis with the bone in continuity results from: an open fracture which has consolidated but with residual infection; direct inoculation of the bone; hematogenous osteomyelitis.

Case report

A 15 year old boy presented with hematogenous osteomyelitis of the distal tibia. Radiographs indicated a lytic lesion with the bone in continuity (Fig. 8.1). Débridement was performed through a straight anterior incision. The lytic area was débrided of grossly infected granulation tissue, packed with PMMA–antibiotic beads and closed over a small drain (Fig. 8.2).

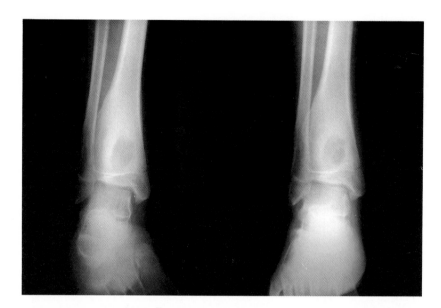

Figure 8.1

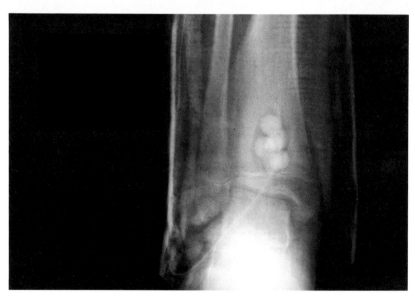

Figure 8.2

Administration of intravenous cefazolin was initiated. Cultures of material obtained intra-operatively were positive for *Staphylococcus aureus*, sensitive to cefazolin. Three weeks after débridement, the beads were removed. Liquefied hematoma was encountered around the beads. The walls of the cavity were covered with healthy granulation tissue. Autogenous cancellous graft was harvested from the iliac crest, mixed with 500 mg vancomycin and used to fill the defect. Systemic cefazolin was continued for an additional three weeks (six weeks total). At five

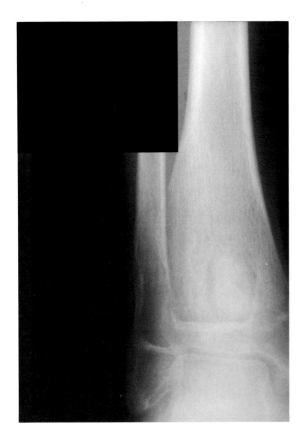

Figure 8.3

months the bone graft appeared to be incorporating and the patient was free of signs and symptoms of infection (Fig. 8.3).

Infected fractures

In the degree of difficulty of management, infected fractures are between focal osteomyelitis with the bone in continuity and infected nonunions. Infected fractures differ from infected nonunions in that there is still potential for the fracture to consolidate. This differs from infected

nonunions in which bony consolidation will not occur without stimulation. There are two techniques of management of infected fractures. The first is immediate débridement of implants and necrotic bone. Stability is achieved with an external fixater. The second technique is to delay débridement until after the fracture has healed. In effect this second alternative is local wound care while waiting for an infected fracture to become focal osteomyelitis with the bone in continuity. I use the second technique in most cases, reserving immediate débridement for two situations: when the infection is aggressive and can only be controlled by systemic antibiotics; or when the implants have failed or loosened and are no longer stabilizing the fracture.

Case report

A 32 year old man sustained a fracture of the calcaneus. Initial management was open reduction and internal fixation via an extensile lateral approach (Fig. 8.4). The tip of the flap sloughed, leaving the plate exposed. Cultures of drainage from the wound were positive for *Pseudomonas aeruginosa*, *Proteus mirabilis*, and *Staphylococcus epidermidis*. Because the plate was holding the reduction and had not loosened, it was left in place. Local wound care consisted of daily whirlpool debridement and twice daily dressing changes. There continued to be a large amount of drainage from the wound; however, cellulitis was absent. The fracture was healed eight weeks after the original surgery (Fig. 8.5), and the plate screws and underlying necrotic bone were removed several weeks later. One screw was buried in viable bone and was left undisturbed. The wound was loosely closed primarily, and systemic antibiotics were initiated and continued for a total of six weeks (Fig. 8.6). Two years following the injury the talocalcaneal articulation has ankylosed and the patient is free of the signs of infections (Fig. 8.7).

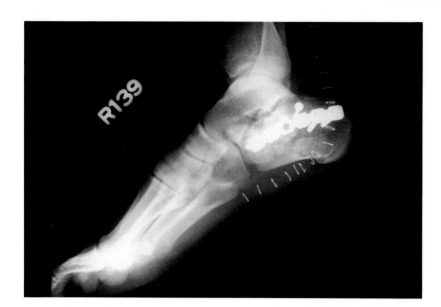

Figure 8.4

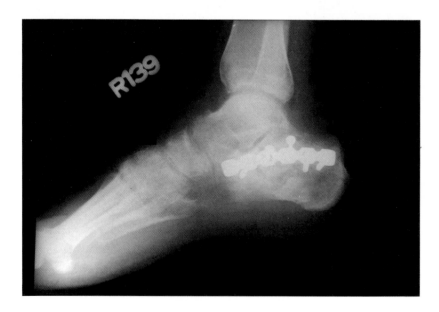

Figure 8.5

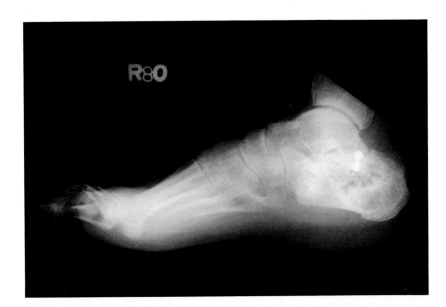

Figure 8.6

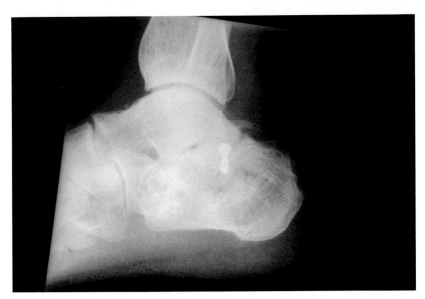

Figure 8.7

Infected nonunion of long bones

Nonunion is defined as an unhealed fracture sustained at least nine months previously with no radiographic or clinical evidence of consolidation in the preceding three months.

The combination of nonunion and infection is a difficult, self-perpetuating problem. The presence of instability exacerbates the symptoms of infection, while the presence of infection makes it less likely that the nonunion will consolidate. Unlike an infected fracture, an infected nonunion has no potential for bony consolidation unless healing is stimulated. Therefore, in addition to addressing instability and infection, the nonunion must be stimulated to consolidate. Stability is achieved with an internal fixation device (plate or nail) or an external fixater (small wire circular frame or rigid large pin uniplanar frames). Antibiotics are administered systemically (intravenously or orally) or locally (via PMMA beads or an implantable pump). Stimulation of healing is achieved by dynamic external fixation, electrical means, or bone grafting. The different methods of antibiotic administration are paired with the different methods of stabilization and the different methods of stimulation depending on the patient's expectations and ability to comply with a management regimen; eg, intravenous administration of antibiotics requires a compliant patient who is able to care for the central line.

Stabilization of infected nonunions

Infected nonunions are stabilized with one of three devices: plates; intramedullary nails; or external fixaters.

Plate

Osteosynthesis is useful in the management of hypertrophic nonunions because fixation is extremely solid. The hypertrophic bone provides excellent purchase for screws. In addition, stimulation of healing is not necessary when the nonunion is hypertrophic because the stability of plate fixation usually results in consolidation without bone grafting. Identification of the pathogenic organisms is necessary prior to plating, so that the appropriate antibiotics can be administered during and after the surgical procedure. Indirect reduction, and limiting subperiosteal dissection to where the plate is applied, minimizes devascularization of the bone. The largest implants possible (eg, broad dynamic

compression plates) are used, to maximize stability.

Case report

A 22 year old man sustained a grade II open tibia fracture, which was managed with débridement and stabilization with an unreamed intramedullary nail (Fig. 8.8). He developed osteomyelitis with drainage from the nail insertion portal and the site of the open fracture. Nine months postinjury, the fracture was thought to be healed, and the nail was removed. The drainage continued, and the patient had persistent pain with weight bearing. Radiographs indicated a probable nonunion (Fig. 8.9). A fibulectomy was performed (Fig. 8.10). Following the fibulectomy, alignment quickly deteriorated, and the nonunion became increasingly hypertrophic (Fig. 8.11). Cultures of the drainage were positive for methicillin resistant *Staphylococcus aureus*. Through a straight anterolateral incision, the nonunion was taken down, alignment was corrected, and a broad dynamic compression plate was applied (Fig. 8.12). No necrotic bone was found; therefore, débridement was minimal. Care was taken not to strip soft tissue from the medial side of the tibia. Bone grafting was not performed. Vancomycin was administered intravenously for six weeks. Cellulitis and drainage quickly subsided; nonweight bearing was continued for three months, at which time there were radiographic signs of consolidation. The patient has been free of signs and symptoms of infection, and is now over 10 years postplating (Fig. 8.13).

Intramedullary nailing

Intramedullary nailing in the management of tibial nonunions has been shown to result in a high incidence of consolidation, low incidence of implant failure, and in addition the patient is allowed to bear weight relatively early in the postoperative period. Another procedure such

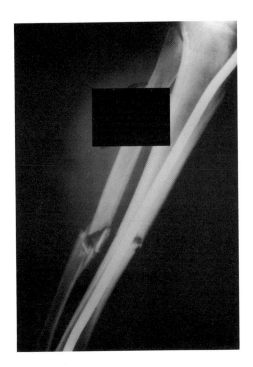

Figure 8.8

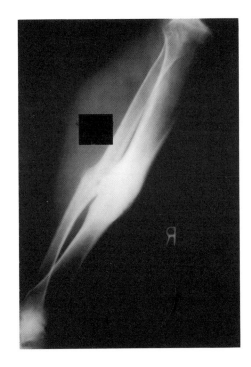

Figure 8.9

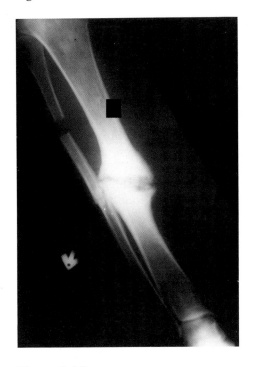

Figure 8.10

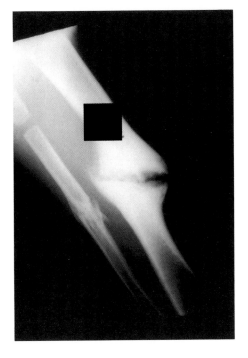

Figure 8.11

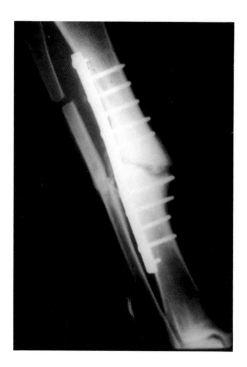

Figure 8.12

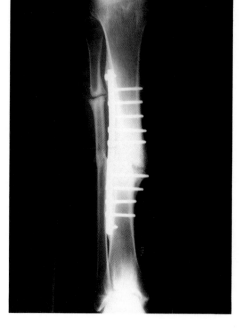

Figure 8.13

as bone grafting, or postoperative manipulation, is not necessary to stimulate healing because the reamings left in the proximity of the nonunion along with the "reinjury" that occurs during reaming and nail insertion are often adequate to stimulate healing. However, the risk of converting localized osteomyelitis to intramedullary osteomyelitis outweighs the advantages and has limited the use of intramedullary nailing in the management of infected nonunions.

Case report

A 28 year old man sustained bilateral grade IIIB open tibial fractures. The fractures were initially managed with débridement, open reduction, and internal fixation with plates. Subsequently, the patient developed osteomyelitis and underwent five débridements, two courses of intravenous antibiotics, and two courses of oral antibiotics. Cultures of drainage were positive for methicillin resistant *Staphylococcus aureus*. At presentation, the patient was nine months post injury. Clinically there was drainage, gross motion at both fracture sites, and the implants were exposed and loose (Figs 8.14–8.16). A pump was inserted to deliver local antibiotics. Both tibias were débrided, the plates were removed, and reamed locked intramedullary nails were inserted. The outflow catheters of the pump were placed in the infected areas. The right tibia drifted into 15° of varus; otherwise, the patient did well (Figs 8.17, 8.18). At three months the area around the outflow catheter in the right leg became erythematous, and shortly thereafter the catheter eroded through the skin (Fig. 8.19). Cultures grew *Staphylococcus*

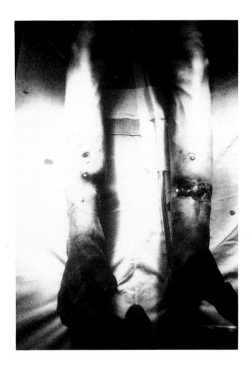

Figure 8.14

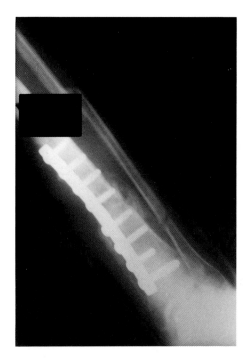

Figure 8.15

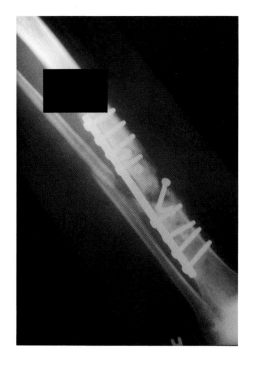

Figure 8.16

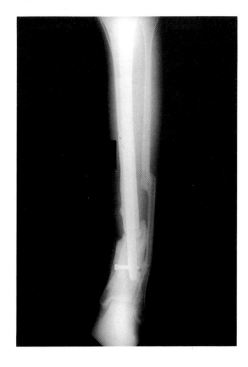

Figure 8.17

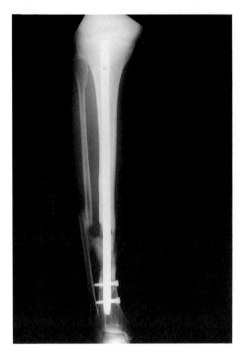

Figure 8.18

epidermidis. The pump and catheters were removed and vancomycin was administered intravenously for two weeks. Six months later, when both nonunions had consolidated the nails were removed and PMMA–antibiotic beads were inserted down the intramedullary canal of the right tibia (Fig. 8.20). Vancomycin was administered for six weeks, for the assumed latent *Staphylococcus epidermidis* infection of the right tibia. The beads were removed three weeks after they had been inserted and the wound closed over a drain. The patient has remained free of infection (Figs 8.21–8.23). He has refused to undergo a corrective osteotomy of the left tibia.

External fixation

External fixation has the theoretical advantage in the management of infected nonunions of providing stability without introduction of a foreign body into the infected area. When an external fixater is used only to stabilize the nonunion,

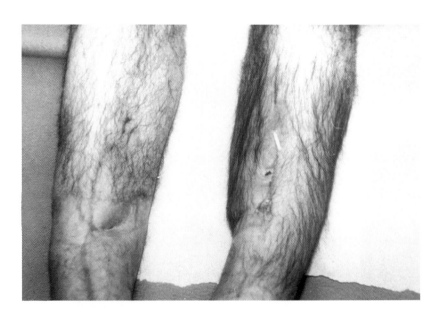

Figure 8.19

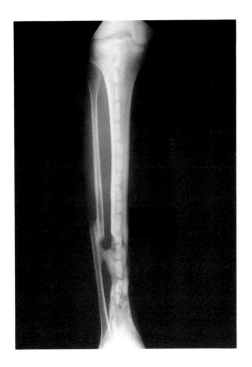

Figure 8.20

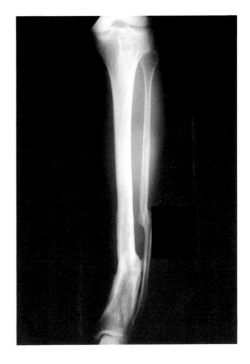

Figure 8.21

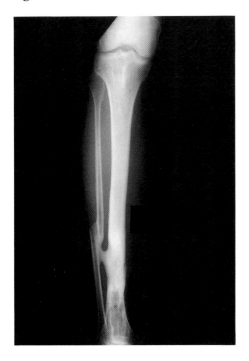

Figure 8.22

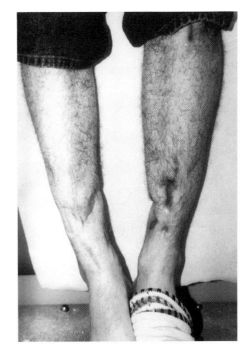

Figure 8.23

healing must be stimulated in order for the non-union to consolidate. This is most frequently accomplished with cancellous grafting. When the external fixater is used not only to stabilize the nonunion, but also to stimulate healing via cyclical compression and distraction (ie, a dynamic external fixater), no further stimulation of healing is required.

Stimulation of infected nonunions

Infected nonunions are stimulated to heal by one of three techniques: dynamic external fixation; electrical means; and autogenous bone grafting.

Dynamic external fixation

Dynamic external fixation has two relative contraindications: nonunions with an oblique configuration, and nonunions that are older than two years. Stimulation of healing is in part due to compression. Nonunions which have an oblique configuration develop shear stresses when compressed. Therefore, there is a high incidence of failure of the nonunion to consolidate when a dynamic external fixater is used to stimulate healing of oblique nonunions. In addition to the architecture of the nonunion, the age of the nonunion is important. There must be some residual capability for consolidation. Very old nonunions seem to have lost this capability and therefore do not heal when managed with dynamic external fixation.

Small wire circular frames are used to manage nonunions that have an associated deformity and periarticular nonunions in which there is not enough bone to insert large pins. Large pin rigid frames are used to manage diaphyseal and metaphyseal nonunions that do not have an associated deformity. Hypertrophic nonunions are managed by cyclically compressing and distracting the nonunion. The rate of compression and distraction is significantly less than that used for

bone transport. A typical schedule is: alternating two week of distraction at 0.25–0.5 mm/day, with one week of compression at the same rate until there is radiographic evidence of healing, at which time compression and distraction are discontinued. Hypotrophic and oligotrophic nonunions are managed with compression alone. An initially rapid rate of compression impacts the bone ends and is followed by a slow rate to maintain compressive forces across the nonunion. A typical schedule is compression at a rate of 1 mm/day for one week followed by 0.25 mm/day on alternate days until there is evidence of consolidation. Weight bearing is encouraged and physical therapy is initiated to improve mobility of neighboring joints. When there is radiographic evidence of consolidation, the frame is dynamized; if the patient continues to bear weight without pain, the frame is removed.

Case report

A 22 year old man had 15 months previously an open distal tibia fracture initially managed with an intramedullary nail. The nail was removed prior to bony healing because of irritation and drainage positive for *Staphylococcus epidermidis* at the knee. At presentation there was a mildly hypertropic oblique nonunion of the distal tibia (Fig. 8.24). A small wire circular frame external fixater was applied because I thought that the small size of the distal fragment precluded the use of a large pin unilateral frame. A fibular osteotomy was performed. The nonunion was initially distracted to regain length, and then cyclically distracted and compressed (Fig. 8.25). Five months after fixater application, length had been restored and there appeared to be calcification within the nonunion site (Fig. 8.26). The frame was discontinued because of patient intolerance. One month after frame removal, the tibia had shortened and angulated (Fig. 8.27). This case illustrates the difficulty of obtaining union

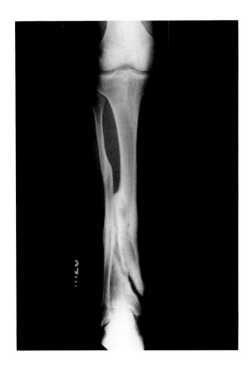

Figure 8.24

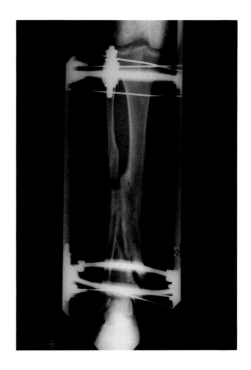

Figure 8.25

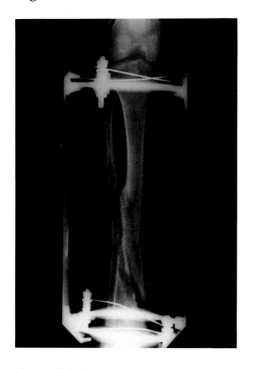

Figure 8.26

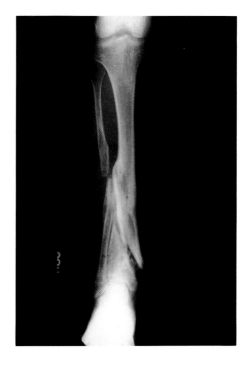

Figure 8.27

with dynamic external fixation in an oblique nonunion.

Case report

A 49 year old man presented 31 years following a midshaft tibia fracture which had resulted in a nonunion. He could bear full weight without pain. His chief complaint was deformity (Figs 8.28, 8.29). There were no signs of infection but there was a clear history of osteomyelitis. A small wire circular frame external fixater was applied and a fibular osteotomy was performed. The varus deformity was corrected, and the nonunion was cyclically distracted and compressed. "Olive" wires were used to obtain additional compression across the nonunion (Fig. 8.30). When consolidation was thought to have occurred at the nonunion site, the fixater was dynamized (ie, the proximal nuts on the side bars were loosened so that weight was borne across the nonunion site). When the patient could bear his full weight without pain, the fixater was removed. At fixater removal, motion at the nonunion site was obvious. The leg was splinted and three weeks later closed intramedullary nailing of the nonunion was performed (Fig. 8.31). Eighteen months after nailing the nonunion is solidly healed (Figs 8.32, 8.33). This case illustrates that cyclical compression and distraction alone are frequently not successful in inducing consolidation of longstanding nonunions.

Case report

A 16 year old male presented one year after a grade III open fracture of the tibia with persistent drainage and pain with weight bearing. Initial treatment of the open fracture had been débridement and external fixation. The peroneal nerve was not functioning; otherwise, the neurovascular examination was within the limits of normal. At presentation, radiographs indicated a hyper-

trophic nonunion, and cultures of drainage were positive for *Staphylococcus aureus* (Figs 8.34, 8.35). The nonunion site was exposed through a straight anterior incision; however, no sequestrum or necrotic tissue was identified. A large pin unilateral dynamic external fixater was applied and the wound was closed (Fig. 8.36). Systemic administration of cefazolin was initiated and continued for six weeks. The nonunion site was cyclically compressed and distracted. The drainage quickly subsided and stopped. The nonunion consolidated and the fixater was removed three months after its application. The patient has remained free of the signs and symptoms of infection (Figs 8.37, 8.38).

Electrical means

Electrical means are used to stimulate consolidation of nonunions when the nonunion is in acceptable alignment, the nonunion gap is less than half the diameter of the bone, and a pseudoarthrosis is not present. Electrical stimulation has the advantage that it is noninvasive; however, débridement and soft tissue coverage may be required after bony consolidation has occurred.

Case report

A 22 year old man presented nine months after a closed tibia fracture. The fracture had been managed with plating. At presentation the plate was exposed (Fig. 8.39), and cultures of drainage grew *Staphylococcus aureus*. Radiographs indicated that the fixation had not loosened. The 7° of varus deformity was considered acceptable (Fig. 8.40). Combined low energy electromagnetic fields were used to stimulate consolidation, local wound care including whirlpool was instituted, and the patient was kept nonweight bearing. Six months later the nonunion had consolidated (Fig. 8.41). A pump was implanted to deliver antibiotics locally, and the plate was removed. The cortex beneath the plate was

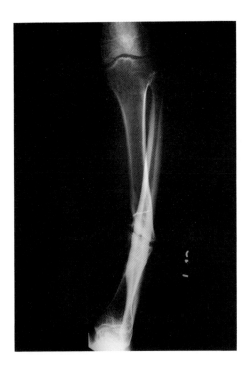

Figure 8.28

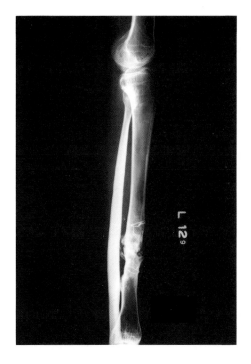

Figure 8.29

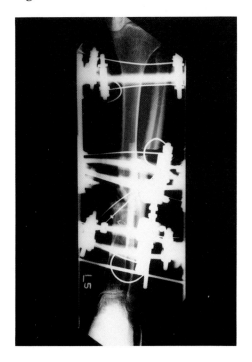

Figure 8.30

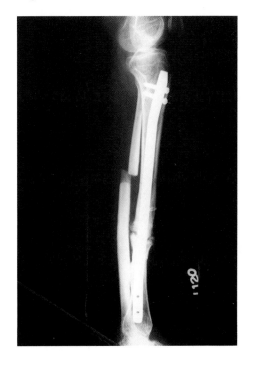

Figure 8.31

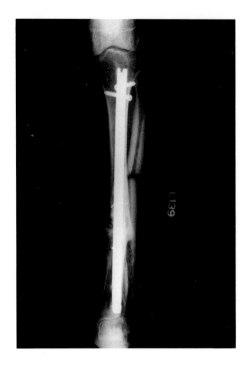

Figure 8.32

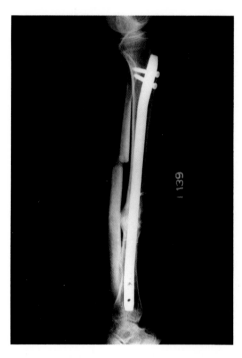

Figure 8.33

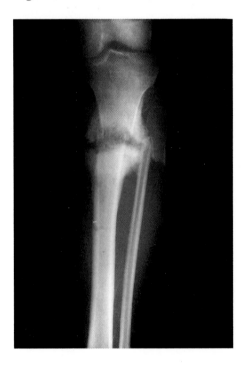

Figure 8.34

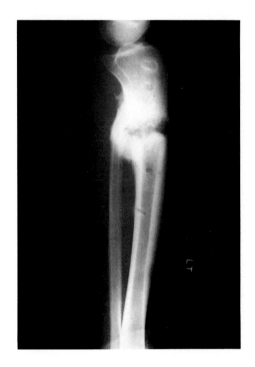

Figure 8.35

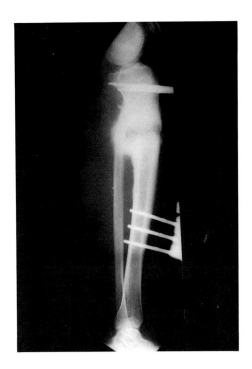

Figure 8.36

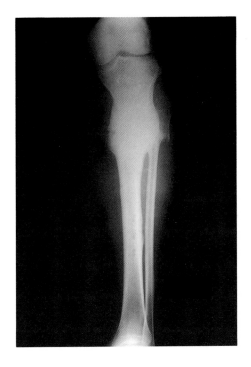

Figure 8.37

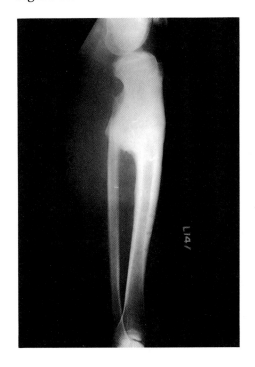

Figure 8.38

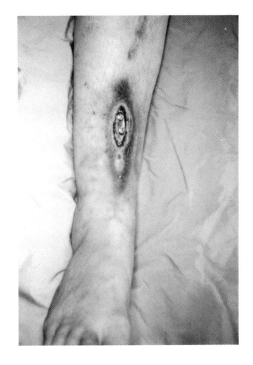

Figure 8.39

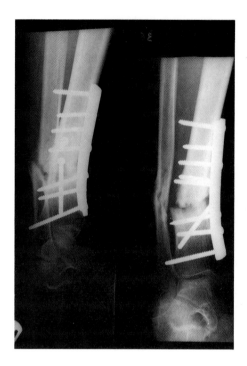

Figure 8.40

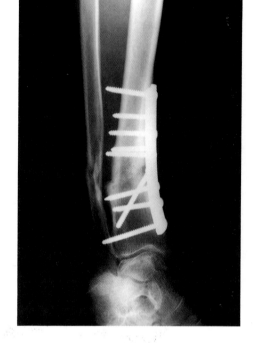

Figure 8.41

necrotic and was débrided. A free tissue transfer was performed to obtain coverage (Fig. 8.42). Antibiotics were administered for a total of eight weeks, at which time the pump was removed. The patient has remained free of infection since surgery (Figs 8.43, 8.44).

Autogenous bone grafting

Autogenous cancellous bone grafting in the management of infected nonunions is combined with a method of stabilization and antibiotic administration. The method of grafting that I find most useful is performed after the focus of infection has been débrided and the wound has been closed primarily or with a soft tissue transfer. PMMA–antibiotic beads are used to maintain the dead space into which the bone graft will

be placed. Antibiotics are administered systemically or locally. At three weeks the wound is opened, and the beads removed. If the cavity appears as though it is no longer infected, cancellous graft is harvested. The graft is mixed with antibiotics and placed in the defect.

Case report

A 48 year old man sustained a grade III open fracture of his distal tibia and fibula. Initial management was débridement and stabilization of the tibia and fibula with a plate and screws (Fig. 8.45). The tibial screws were subsequently removed, and the leg was immobilized in a splint. The patient presented 10 months after injury with a hypertrophic nonunion of the distal tibia in approximately 30° of varus (Fig. 8.46). A

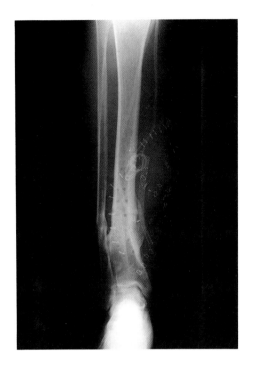

Figure 8.42

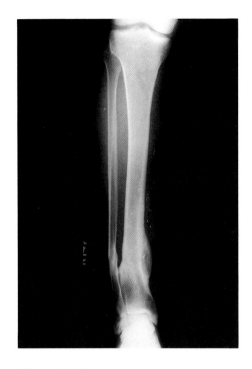

Figure 8.43

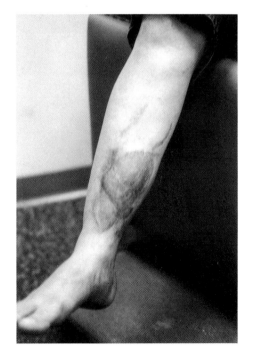

Figure 8.44

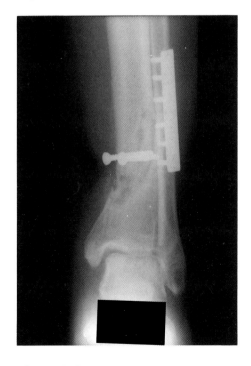

Figure 8.45

draining sinus was present on the medial side of the ankle. Material from the sinus was culture positive for *Escherichia coli* and *Staphylococcus aureus*. The plate was removed from the fibula and the fibula was osteotomized. The nonunion was débrided, the tibial deformity was corrected through the nonunion, and the correction was maintained with an external fixater. The skin was closed primarily. Beads were not used because there was not enough space for them (Figs 8.47, 8.48). Systemic antibiotics were initiated after material for culture had been obtained. Three weeks later autogenous cancellous bone was harvested from the distal femur, mixed with 500 mg vancomycin, and placed in the defect. Systemic antibiotics were continued for an additional three weeks. The cellulitis and drainage quickly resolved and radiographically the nonunion appeared to consolidate (Fig. 8.49). At four months the fixater was dynamized, and there was no increase with pain on weight bearing. The fixater was subsequently removed (Figs 8.50, 8.51) The patient has remained asymptomatic.

Infected segmental defects of long bones

Segmental defects are most frequently the result of an open fracture with loss of bone at the time of injury, or the result of débridement of infected and necrotic bone. These patients invariably have a history of infection. In cases which are not actively infected, one should assume that latent osteomyelitis is present. In some cases shortening of the extremity has decreased the actual size of the segmental defect. Mechanical instability, inadequate soft tissue coverage, local hypovascularity and dead space are present. Stability is achieved with plates, nails, or external fixaters. Inadequate soft tissue coverage, local hypovascularity, and dead space are eliminated with tissue

transfer, PMMA–antibiotic beads, and autogenous cancellous bone graft. Reconstruction of the bony defect is not only essential, but is also the goal which is most challenging to achieve. Reconstruction of the bony defect is achieved with vascularized bone transfer, autogenous cancellous bone graft, or dynamic external fixation. In addition to surgical management, antibiotic administration is required.

Stability: segmental defects

Stability is achieved with plates, intramedullary nails, or external fixaters. The use of plates to stabilize segmental defects is limited by three factors: plates are load bearing and thus fail relatively quickly; the rate of failure is accelerated by the osteopenia associated with segmental defects and the resulting decrease in stability of fixation; and the plate may act as a foreign body and exacerbate preexisting infection. Of these three factors the most serious is the rate of plate failure. An extended period of time is necessary before reconstruction of the bony defect will result in intrinsic stability. This period of time is almost always greater than the life of the plate. Intramedullary nails share the disadvantage of acting as a foreign body and, in addition, they run the risk of converting localized osteomyelitis into intramedullary osteomyelitis. However, they are load sharing, and therefore have a lower rate of failure than plates. Their use is limited to diaphyseal and metadiaphyseal defects. Because of the lower rate of failure, I consider nails a better option than plates. External fixaters can be used in two ways: simply to stabilize the bone without introducing a foreign body into the infected area; or to stabilize the bone and to reconstruct the bony defect. These techniques have been described in the previous section.

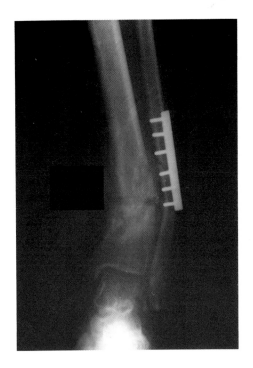

Figure 8.46

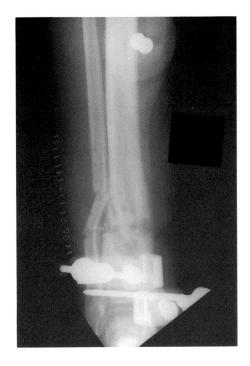

Figure 8.47

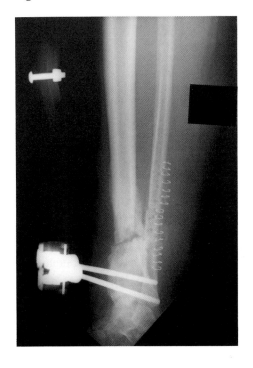

Figure 8.48

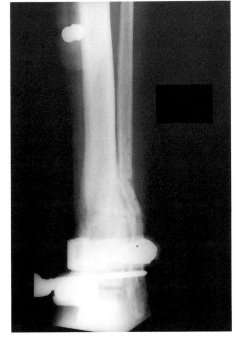

Figure 8.49

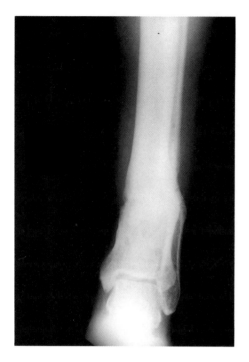

Figure 8.50

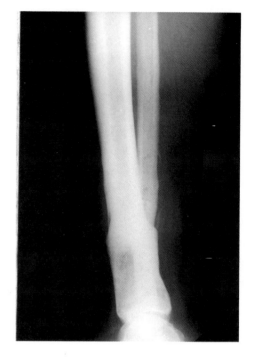

Figure 8.51

Reconstruction: segmental defect

Reconstruction of the bony defect is achieved by autogenous cancellous grafting, free vascularized transfer of bone, or dynamic external fixation.

Autogenous cancellous bone grafting is the oldest method of management of segmental defects. The technique is very simple, but the duration of treatment can be prolonged.

Case report

A 39 year old man presented nine months after a grade III segmental tibia fracture. The fracture had been initially managed with débridement and fixation with interfragmental screws and an external fixater. The external fixater had been subsequently removed. On presentation there was exposed bone proximally and gross motion at both fractures (Figs 8.52, 8.53). Cultures of wound drainage grew *Staphylococcus aureus* and a number of Gram negative rods. The tibia was débrided through a straight anterior incision. At surgery, the entire intercalary segment of bone was found to be necrotic and was removed. An external fixater was applied and the dead space was packed with PMMA–antibiotic beads (Figs 8.54, 8.55). The wound was closed primarily over a large drain. Three weeks later the beads were removed and cancellous bone from both iliac crests was mixed with 1 g vancomycin and used to fill the dead space. In addition, the proximal and distal tibial syndesmoses were fused (Fig. 8.56). Systemic antibiotics were administered for a total of six weeks. Another bone graft was

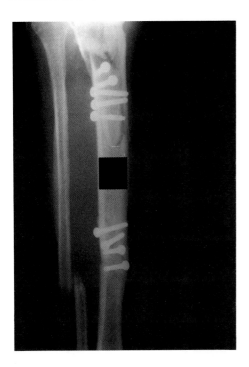

Figure 8.52

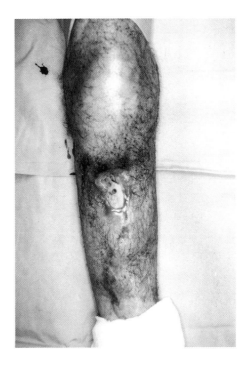

Figure 8.53

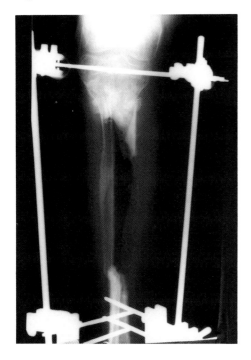

Figure 8.54

performed three months after the initial surgery. The graft slowly consolidated, and at one year the fixater was removed. Nonweight bearing was maintained until the graft had hypertrophied. At 20 months full weight bearing was initiated (Fig. 8.57). The patient subsequently sustained a stress fracture through the graft, and has had one episode of cellulitis which responded to oral antibiotics; otherwise, he has done well (Figs 8.58, 8.59).

Vascularized bone transfer

Vascularized bone transfers have two theoretical advantages: when a vascularized block of bone is transferred, it imparts mechanical stability to the extremity; and there is a decreased incidence of nonunion or delayed nonunion within the bone graft itself. A segment of bone (fibula or iliac crest) is only transferred because it is vascularized, viable, and, therefore, somewhat resistant

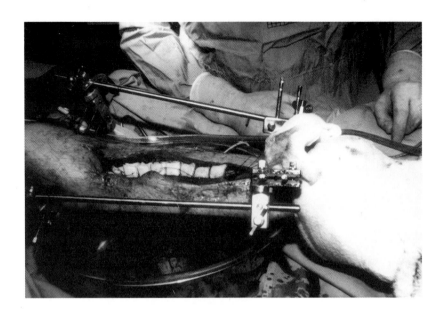

Figure 8.55

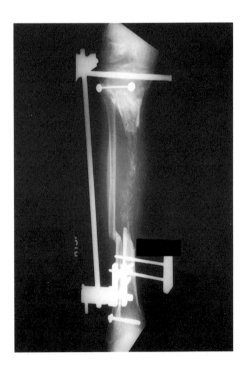

Figure 8.56

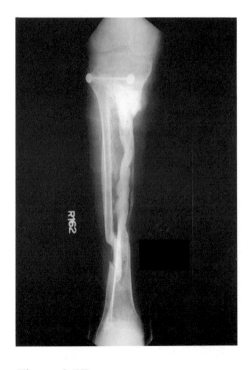

Figure 8.57

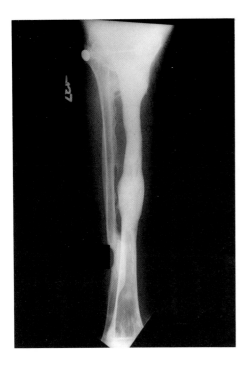

Figure 8.58

to infection. A segment of avascular, or necrotic, bone should never be transferred into an infected segmental defect.

Case report

A 28 year old man sustained a Grade III open tibia fracture in an automobile accident. Initial management was débridement and stabilization with a large pin external fixater. Two months after the original injury the patient had well healed incisions, good soft tissue coverage, and an 8 cm gap in the mid-diaphyseal tibia. The fixater was still in place (Fig. 8.60). A free vascularized fibula was harvested from the opposite extremity, and used to bridge the gap. The vascular anastomosis was with the anterior tibial artery. The transferred fibula was split to encourage hypertrophy, and its ends were stabilized to the tibia with screws and wires. The fibular–tibial junctions were bone grafted with autogenous cancellous graft. At six months the fixater frame was modified by removing the medial bar, leaving only the anterior bar and two pins above

Figure 8.59

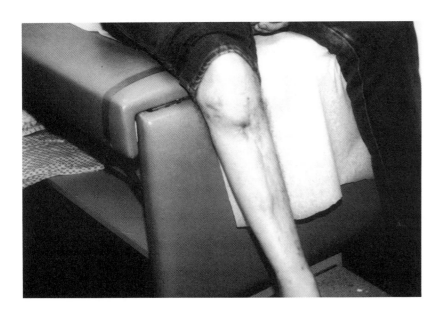

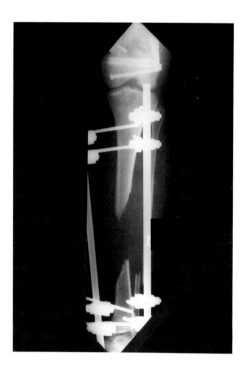

Figure 8.60

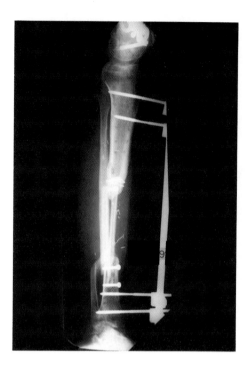

Figure 8.61

and below the segmental defect (Fig. 8.61). Three months later the proximal and distal graft sites appeared to have consolidated (Fig. 8.62). The fixater was removed and weight bearing was initiated. Two years following the initial injury the free fibula is solidly healed to the tibia and the patient is full weight bearing, with no signs of infection (Fig. 8.63).

Dynamic external fixator

Dynamic external fixators can be used to reconstruct segmental defects of any long bone; however, most of our experience is with the tibia. The fixater is used to manipulate fragments of osteotomized bone slowly in such a way that the defect fills in with new, or regenerate, bone. The two basic types of external fixater used to manage segmental defects are rigid large pin uniplanar frames, and flexible small wire circular ring frames. A description of these frames and

their uses and advantages is found in Chapter 6. In general, uniplanar frames are used when deformity is not present, and on bones other than the tibia. Circular frames are used primarily on the tibia when there is deformity.

Case report

A 58 year old man sustained a grade III open tibia fracture when his leg was crushed in a grain auger. Initial management was débridement and fixation with a broad dynamic compression plate and screws. He subsequently developed osteomyelitis and presented with the plate exposed (Figs 8.64, 8.65). Cultures of drainage from the wound grew methicillin resistant *Staphylococcus aureus*. The plate and screws were removed, and the tibia was débrided, resulting in a segmental defect. Stability was achieved with an external fixater (Fig. 8.66). A free latissimus dorsi transfer was performed and the

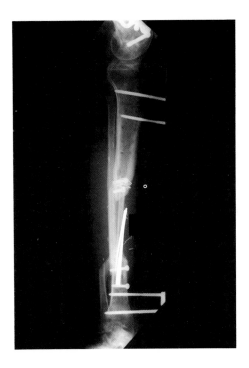

Figure 8.62

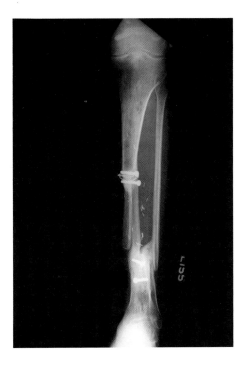

Figure 8.63

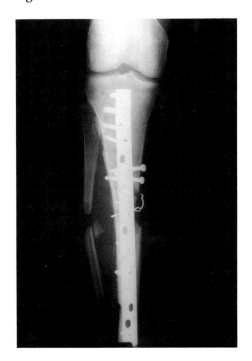

Figure 8.64

defect was packed with PMMA–antibiotic beads. Three weeks after the tissue transfer, a small wire circular frame was applied, and a corticotomy was performed at the distal metaphysis. Two weeks after bone transport had been initiated, the beads were removed (Fig. 8.67). The docking site did not consolidate; therefore, a plate was applied and the site was bone grafted (Fig. 8.68). The patient did well for three years, after which time he developed an abscess over the plate. Cultures were positive for methicillin resistant *Staphylococcus aureus*, the original pathogen. The plate was removed, and systemic antibiotics were administered for six weeks. Cellulitis and drainage quickly resolved, and the patient has been free of the signs and symptoms of infection since this last incision and drainage (Fig. 8.69).

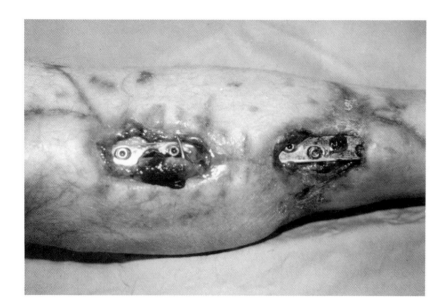

Figure 8.65

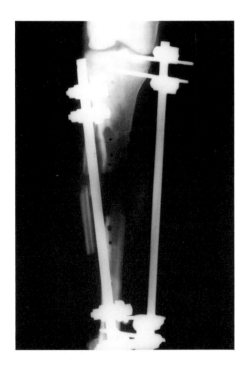

Figure 8.66

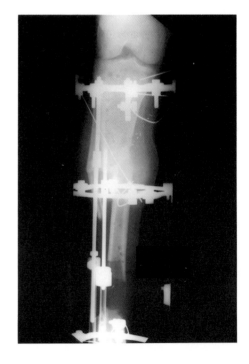

Figure 8.67

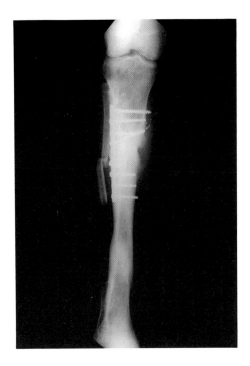

Figure 8.68

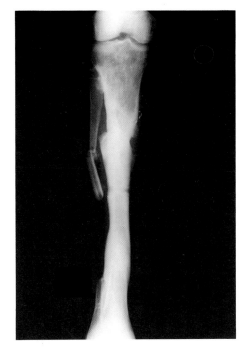

Figure 8.69

Nonunion with latent osteomyelitis

Patients with a nonunion and a history of infection are at risk of reactivation of their infection when their nonunion is managed operatively. Plating of a nonunion has the advantage that deformity can be corrected. However, it has the disadvantage of an increased chance of activating a latent infection when an extensive dissection is required and a large implant is left in the wound. Nailing of nonunions with latent infection has the advantage that the patient can bear weight early in the postoperative period. Nailing has the disadvantage that it is associated with a high incidence of activation of infection. When this occurs the infection often spreads proximally and distally along the nail, involving the entire medullary canal.

Our method of choice in the management of nonunions with latent infection is a dynamic external fixater and stimulation of healing with cyclical distraction and compression. Indications for open reduction and plating of a nonunion are: a displaced intraarticular nonunion; and when removal of a plate and screws is necessary. Because of the high incidence of flare up, we seldom nail nonunions with a latent infection.

Case report

A 19 year old man sustained a grade III open tibia fracture. Initial management was débridement, and stabilization with an external fixater. A postinjury wound infection developed and cultures of material obtained from the wound were positive for *Staphylococcus aureus*. A latissimus dorsi transfer provided soft tissue coverage, and antibiotics were administered systemically for six weeks. The external fixater was removed six months after injury because of inflammation around the pin tracts. The patient presented nine months after injury. The incisions had healed, and there was no drainage or other signs of infection. The patient used a removable short leg splint; however, weight bearing was painful and motion at the nonunion was clinically apparent (Fig. 8.70). The nonunion was biopsied. Material obtained from the biopsy failed to grow any organisms. A closed intramedullary nailing was performed. (Fig. 8.71). Systemic antibiotics were administered for two days following surgery. The patient did well for three weeks, after which the leg became swollen, painful, and fluid began to drain from the nail insertion site. Radiographs obtained five weeks after nailing indicated osteolysis around the entire length of the nail and disorganized new bone formation (Fig. 8.72). Cultures were positive for *Staphylococcus aureus*. Daily whirlpool débridement and twice daily dressing changes were initiated. The swelling and pain and drainage slowly decreased as the nonunion began to consolidate. At six months the incisions had healed and the nonunion had consolidated (Fig. 8.73). The patient refused to undergo another procedure to remove the nail and has been lost to follow up. This case illustrates activation of latent osteomyelitis following intramedullary nailing of a nonunion.

Case report

An 83 year old woman presented eight months after a low energy bicondylar tibial plateau fracture. Initial management was open reduction and stabilization with a plate. Postoperatively, the patient had drainage from the wound, which grew *Pseudomonas* when cultured. After four weeks of intravenous antibiotics the drainage had stopped. At presentation the incisions were well healed and radiographs indicated loss of fixation and varus deformity (Fig. 8.74). Management consisted of removal of the implants, realignment of the nonunion, autogenous bone grafting from the ipsilateral distal femur, and stabilization with new plates (Fig. 8.75). The bone graft with mixed with 1 g vancomycin, and postoperatively intravenous antibiotics were administered for four weeks. This case illustrates management of a nonunion with latent osteomyelitis with plates, bone graft, and systemic and local antibiotics.

Case report

A 28 year old man sustained a grade II open fracture of the humeral diaphysis. Initial management was débridement and stabilization with retrograde flexible intramedullary nails. The patient developed cellulitis around the site of the open fracture, and cultures of the drainage were positive for *Staphylococcus aureus*. Systemic antibiotics were administered for six weeks, and cellulitis and drainage resolved; however, the fracture site remained painful. Radiographs obtained nine months after injury indicated nonunion (Fig. 8.76). Ten months after injury the flexible nails were removed, the humerus was reamed and stabilized with a rigid antegrade nail. Postoperatively there were no signs of activation of the infection; however, the patient continued to have pain at the nonunion site. Radiographs obtained eight months after antegrade nailing indicated a persistent nonunion (Fig. 8.77). The nail was removed and a large pin unilateral dynamic fixater was applied (Fig. 8.78). The patient applied compression across the nonunion initially at the rate of 1 mm per day. When it was clear that the bone ends were in contact, cyclical compression and distraction were initiated. The frame was removed one year after its application when the nonunion had consolidated (Fig. 8.79).

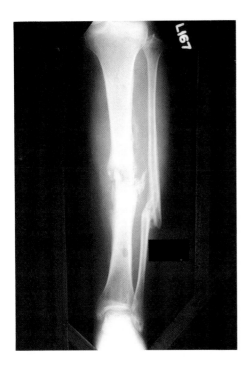

Figure 8.70

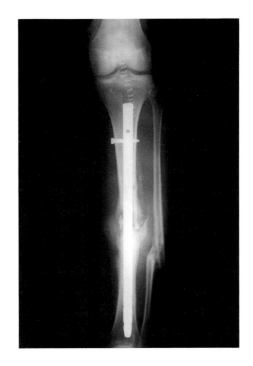

Figure 8.71

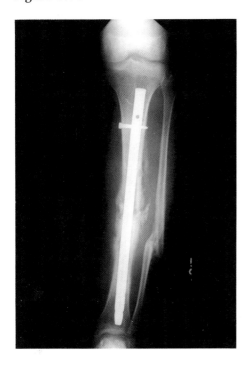

Figure 8.72

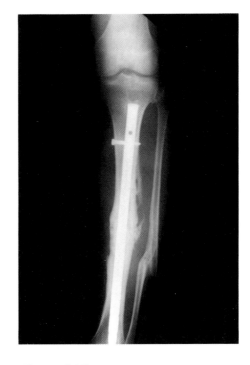

Figure 8.73

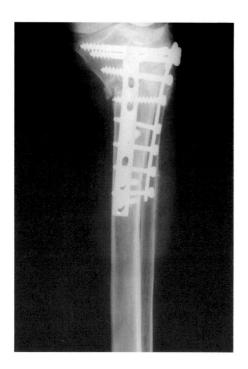

Figure 8.74

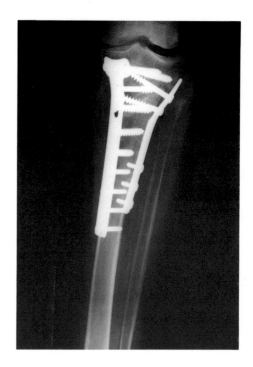

Figure 8.75

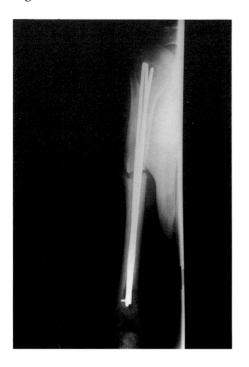

Figure 8.76

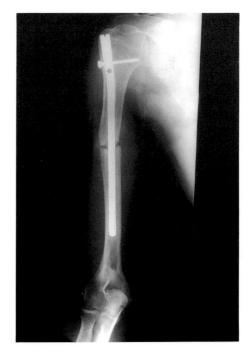

Figure 8.77

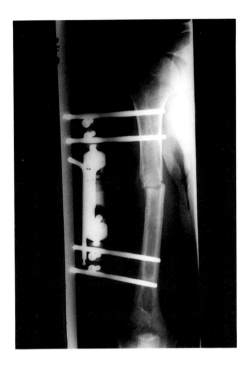

Figure 8.78

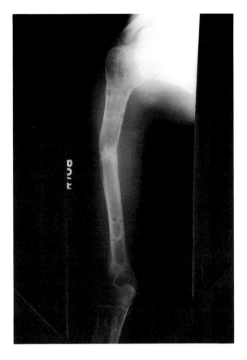

Figure 8.79

Infection of lower extremity in the diabetic patient

The principles of management of the infected lower extremity in the diabetic patient are similar to those of osteomyelitis (ie, débridement, coverage, stabilization, and dead space management), with several exceptions and caveats. The microcirculation of the extremity is compromised; therefore, healing will be slower. Débridement of bone may concentrate stress on other areas of the foot, speeding their breakdown (eg, débridement of the fourth and fifth metatarsals increases the load on the first, second and third metatarsals). It is important to maintain the patient's ability to bear weight on the extremity, as the other foot may also become involved, and bilateral amputees are often confined to a wheel-

chair. This group of patients is frequently malnourished; therefore it is extremely important to establish the nutritional status and, if indicated, to improve it. Management is based upon the grade of infection.

Grade 0 infections, ie, the skin is intact with underlying bony deformity, are managed by trimming calluses and nails, modifying footwear to relieve areas of increased pressure, and educating the patient and his or her family.

Grade 1 and 2 infections are those which involve only partial thickness of the skin, or full thickness of the skin, but do not involve tendon or bone. These infections are managed initially with local débridement. Invariably, there is cellulitis associated with the ulcer. Material from the débridement is sent for culture, and broad spectrum systemic antibiotics are administered. It is important not to administer antibiotics until the débridement has been performed. These infections are usually polymicrobial, and the pathogens are resistant to commonly utilized antibiotics; therefore, intravenous administration of potentially toxic antibiotics is necessary. Two to seven days following débridement, when it is clear that the wound has stabilized, a total contact cast is applied. Nonweight bearing is maintained for the first several weeks. At two to four weeks the cast is changed, and if the wound appears to be healing, weight is increased as tolerated. Antibiotic therapy is discontinued when the cellulitis subsides, at a minimum of 10 days. As long as the wound improves, casting is continued with cast changes every two to four weeks, until the wound is healed. An alternative to total contact casting is to institute a program of daily or twice daily dressing changes. Nonweight bearing is maintained until the wound is healthy enough to skin graft.

Grade 3 infections are ulcers which extend through the skin and involve bone and tendons. These infections are managed by extensive débridement in the operating room of all necrotic tissue. Frequently, more than one operative débridement is required. Removal of bony prominences, dead space management, coverage with free tissue transfers, and antibiotic administration are potentially useful techniques of management.

A grade 4 infection denotes necrosis of the toes or entire forefoot. Patients with an ankle arm index of greater than 0.45 are managed with an amputation through the foot. The precise level of the amputation depends on the extent and location of necrosis. Amputations of one or more toes, one or two rays, the forefoot through Chopart's joint, and of the entire foot preserving the heel pad (Syme's amputation) have been successful. In cases in which the ankle arm index is less than 0.45, a below knee amputation is performed, with the understanding that it may have to be revised to a knee disarticulation or above knee amputation.

Grade 5 infection denotes necrosis of the entire foot. Management is amputation. The level of the amputation depends upon the extent of necrosis; if possible, the knee is salvaged. As in grade 4 infections, an ankle arm index of less than 0.45 indicates a poor prognosis for a below knee amputation, but by itself does not contraindicate an attempt to salvage the knee.

Acute septic arthritis

The method of management of a septic joint is determined by whether the infection is acute or chronic, and by the identity of the pathogenic organisms. The first step in the management of a patient presenting with a possible acute or subacute joint infection is aspiration of the joint. Aspiration is both therapeutic and diagnostic. It is therapeutic because it temporarily decompresses the joint and decreases symptoms. The material obtained is cultured, a cell count and Gram stain are obtained, and the fluid is examined for crystals. The second step is administration of systemic antibiotics. Antibiotics are initiated because the sooner the infection is controlled, the less damage there is to intraarticular structures. The risk is that the material obtained by aspiration will be sterile, and that the more definitive intraoperative cultures will also be negative because of the antibiotics.

Acute septic arthritis in which there is a high index of suspicion that the causal organism is *Gonococcus* or Lyme disease and in which the synovial fluid cell count is less than 75,000/ml are managed with aspiration and antibiotic therapy. In cases in which a clear decrease in symptoms does not occur within 24 hours of initiation of antibiotic therapy, the joint is incised and drained, and fragments of synovium are cultured. In equivocal cases the joint is reaspirated and the synovial fluid cell count is determined. If there has not been a significant decrease in the cell count relative to the initial aspiration, the joint is incised and drained.

Acute septic arthritis caused by Gram positive aerobic organisms and *Haemophilus influenzae* are managed with arthrotomy, débridement, closure over drains, and four weeks of systemic antibiotics. I use repeated aspiration only when the patient is too ill to undergo a surgical procedure, or multiple joints are involved.

Acute septic arthritis caused by Gram negative aerobes are managed with arthrotomy, débridement, and closure over drains. Because infections caused by Gram negative aerobes are more likely to recur, I have a low threshold for surgical reexploration and administering antibiotics for longer than four weeks.

Infections caused by anaerobic organisms are rare and occur in immune suppressed patients. These organisms are frequently very sensitive to antibiotics, and because frequently the patients medical condition precludes surgery, repeated aspiration is used to drain the joint.

Acute septic arthritis caused by mycobacterial and fungal organisms is extremely rare, presenting most frequently in the chronic stage. Management consists of arthrotomy and extensive débridement, including synovectomy and curettage of periarticular cysts. Usually, the articular surfaces of the joint are destroyed. Therefore, the joint is immobilized in a position of function, in anticipation of ankylosis.

Chronic septic arthritis

Chronic septic arthritis is the result of neglected or unsuccessfully managed acute septic arthritis. Regardless of its stage, management begins with arthrotomy, synovectomy and closure over tubes. In cases in which there is associated osteomyelitis, intraosseous abscesses and necrotic bone are débrided. The extremity is immobilized in a position of function (knees at 10°, hips in traction in 0° of abduction and 30° of flexion, and elbows in 90° of flexion and 20° of supination). Appropriate systemic antibiotics are

administered for six weeks. In cases in which reconstruction is required, it is performed at a later date, a minimum of three months following the conclusion of antibiotic therapy.

Case report

A 54 year old man underwent outpatient arthroscopy for internal derangement of the knee. Postoperatively, he had more swelling and pain than expected. Five days after the initial procedure, the knee was aspirated and 40 ml of turbid fluid was obtained. Specimens were sent for cell count and culture. While the results were pending the patient was started on oral cephalexin. The cell count was 30,000/ml and the cultures were positive, in broth only, for *Staphylococcus epidermidis*. The positive culture was considered to be the result of skin contamination; nevertheless, oral antibiotics were continued. Three weeks after the arthroscopy, the effusion had reaccumulated and pain and loss of motion were increasing. Arthroscopic débridement was performed, and intravenous cefazolin was initiated. Cultures of material obtained at arthroscopy were positive again for *Staphylococcus epidermidis*. The cefazolin was discontinued, and vancomycin was administered for two weeks, followed by ciprofloxacin for two weeks. The effusion recurred when the ciprofloxacin was discontinued. The patient presented 10 weeks after the initial arthroscopy. The knee was swollen with a "boggy" effusion, and the range of motion was severely limited; radiographs indicated loss of joint space, with no obvious periarticular cysts, or signs of osteomyelitis (Figs 8.80, 8.81). A radical synovectomy was performed through a midline incision. The capsule and synovium were edematous and hypertrophic. (Fig. 8.82). Closer inspection of the femoral condyle (Fig. 8.83) revealed hypertrophic synovium (black arrow) and pannus (white arrow) overgrowing the articular cartilage of the femoral condyle ("C"). Synovium and scarred capsule were excised, increasing the range of motion of

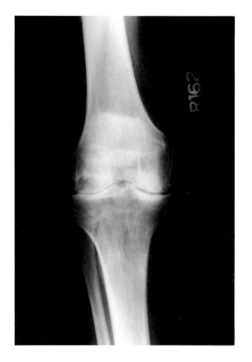

Figure 8.80

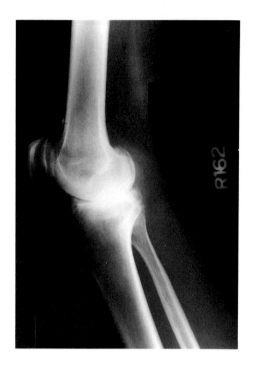

Figure 8.81

Figure 8.82

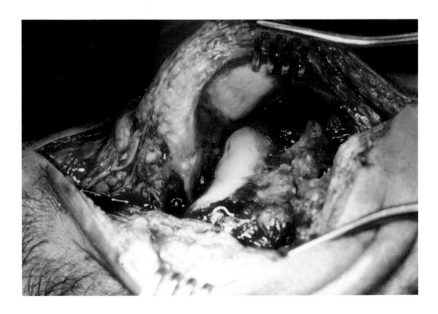

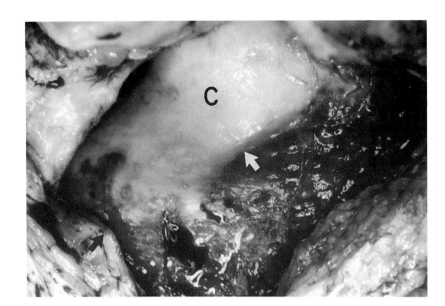

Figure 8.83

the knee. Closure was over large suction drains. Continuous passive motion was initiated post-operatively, and utilized for four weeks, while the patient slept. Vancomycin was administered systemically for six weeks. While there were no further indications of infection, the patient did have persistent pain with motion and weight bearing. Six months following the final débridement, a total joint arthroplasty was performed (Fig. 8.84). The patient has done well, with no further signs of infection (Figs 8.85, 8.86).

Infection in a patient with a hemaglobinopathy

When a patient with a hemaglobinopathy has the acute onset of pain, the primary differential diagnosis is between infection and bone infarct.[1,2] The patient is admitted. An internist or pediatrician with specific interest in the management of patients with hemaglobinopathies is consulted. The patient is hydrated and the extremity is

splinted. Radiographs are obtained. Based upon the radiographs and the physical examination, suspected areas of infection are aspirated prior to antibiotic administration. If any material is obtained it is sent for culture and Gram stain, and antibiotics are administered. In cases in which the Gram stain indicates Gram positive cocci, an antistaphylococcal antibiotic (eg, cephalothin) is administered. In cases in which the gram stain indicates gram negative rods, an antisalmonella antibiotic (eg, ampicillin or chloramphenicol) is administered. When the Gram stain is negative, both *Staphylococcus aureus* and *Salmonella* are covered until cultures are positive. Open biopsy is avoided whenever possible. Blood cultures are obtained; if positive they indicate that there is an active infection and they identify the pathogen. Stool cultures are obtained specifically for *Salmonella*. If the patient is infected, the presence of *Salmonella* in the stool is associated with a high probability that *Salmonella* is the pathogen, and the appropriate antibiotic therapy is started.

The next step is to rule out bone infarct as the cause of symptoms. Tc-99, Ga-67, or In-111 scans are obtained. Increased uptake on the

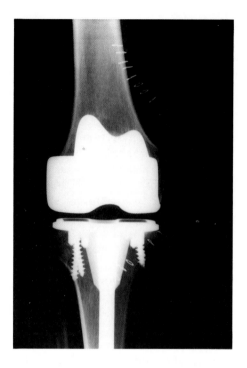

Figure 8.84

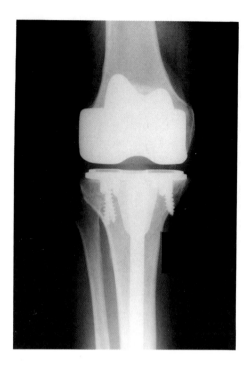

Figure 8.85

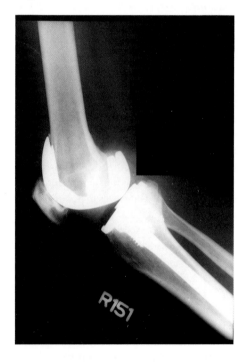

Figure 8.86

delayed Tc-99 and Ga-67 or the In-111 scan indicate infection. Decreased uptake on any of the scans indicates a bone infarct. In addition, the scans are examined for occult areas of infection. An elevated erythrocyte sedimentation rate and white blood cell count do not help differentiate infection from infarct.

When the diagnosis of infection is made, the patient is prepared for surgery by exchange transfusion to raise the level of hemoglobin A to over 60%, and hydration to minimize sickling due to increased viscosity. Intraoperatively, tourniquets are never used. All abscesses are drained, and necrotic tissue débrided. Intramedullary abscesses are identified by drilling through the cortex. If present, they are unroofed. Wounds are closed over large drains. In cases in which the bone has been weakened significantly by débridement, autogenous cancellous bone grafting is performed at three to six weeks.

Infected arthroplasties

Our management of infected total joint arthroplasties follows one of four basic pathways: long term suppression, with retention of the prosthesis; débridement and local antibiotic administration, with retention of the prosthesis; exchange arthroplasty; or removal of the prosthesis without reimplantation.

Long term suppression

Long term suppression is indicated when the patient's symptoms do not warrant an exchange arthroplasty. In general, this method of management is used for low demand patients or patients in whom an exchange arthroplasty has failed and whose symptoms are controlled with oral antibiotics. Oral antibiotics are administered with the understanding that the infection is not cured and that periprosthetic lysis may progress, making reimplantation of a prosthesis more difficult. Chronic drainage is unacceptable, as it frequently leads to infection with resistant, more invasive pathogens. Therefore, chronic drainage is an indication for more aggressive therapy.

Case report

A 64 year old man underwent total knee arthroplasty for osteoarthritis. Postoperatively, a circumferential partial thickness skin slough developed around the thigh, corresponding to the location of the tourniquet. Because of this skin loss, systemic antibiotics were administered postoperatively. The incision did not heal as expected and continued to drain small amounts of clear fluid. The partial thickness skin loss around the thigh epithelialized with dressing changes. Six weeks after surgery, fluid from the incision was cultured and grew *Staphylococcus aureus*. On presentation, the patient's knee was erythematous and slightly swollen; the central third of the incision had dehisced and was draining purulent fluid. There were no radiographic signs of bone–prosthesis interface involvement. A pump was implanted, and the knee débrided, leaving the prosthesis in situ. The outflow catheters from the pump were placed in the knee, which was closed over large suction drains (Fig. 8.87). The signs and symptoms of infection resolved almost immediately, and at seven weeks the pump was removed. Within four weeks the patient developed recurrent swelling and pain. Aspiration of the knee yielded purulent material which was positive for *Staphylococcus aureus*, sensitive to cephalosporins. Oral cephalexin was initiated, and the patient was scheduled for removal of the prosthesis and débridement of the knee. The pain and swelling resolved prior to surgery and the patient elected not to undergo the scheduled operation. Radiographs obtained three and four years after arthroplasty indicate lucency around the components (Figs 8.88, 8.89). Six years following arthroplasty the patient continues to be active, with minimal symptoms related to the knee.

Débridement and antibiotic administration

Débridement and antibiotic administration with retention of the prosthesis are indicated when there are no signs of involvement of the bone–prosthesis interface. We attempt to salvage the prosthesis with débridement and local antibiotic administration via an implantable pump. The prosthesis is left in situ only when it is in good position, the duration of infection is less than six weeks, and there is no radiographic evidence of periprosthetic lysis.

Case report

A 68 year old woman underwent total knee arthroplasty. Postoperatively, her wound dehisced and she developed a wound infection. Cultures were positive for *Staphylococcus*

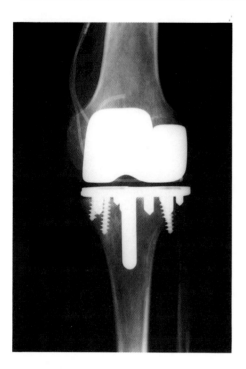

Figure 8.87

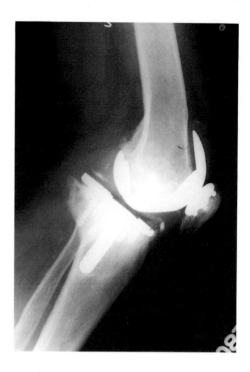

Figure 8.88

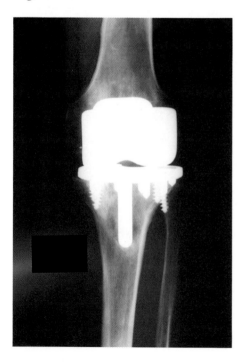

Figure 8.89

aureus. Four weeks after the arthroplasty a pump was implanted and the knee was opened and drained. Careful examination of the components revealed no evidence of infection of the bone–prosthesis interface. The outflow catheters of the pump were placed in the knee, and the knee was closed over large suction drains (Figs 8.90, 8.91). Cellulitis and swelling resolved. Three months later the pump was removed as an outpatient procedure. One of the outflow catheters broke off in the joint, and was left behind. The patient is now four years posttherapy and continues to do well (Figs 8.92, 8.93).

Exchange arthropasty

Exchange arthroplasty is performed in cases in which the arthroplasty has been infected for more than six weeks, or in which there are radiographic signs of involvement of the bone–prothesis interface. The prosthesis is removed

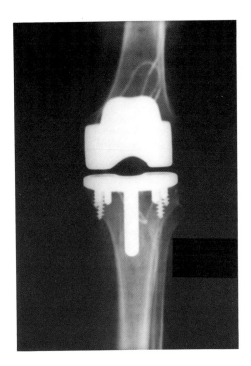

Figure 8.90

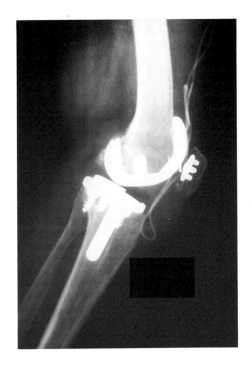

Figure 8.91

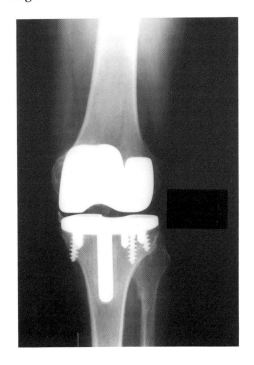

Figure 8.92

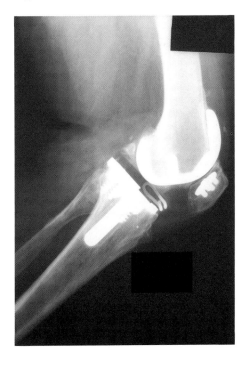

Figure 8.93

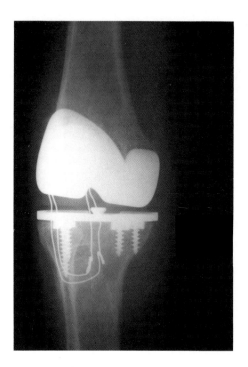

Figure 8.94

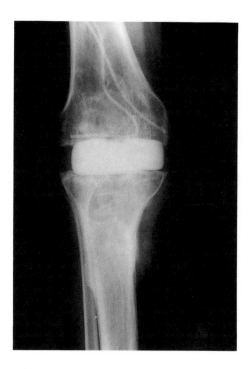

Figure 8.95

along with any cement and necrotic tissue. A PMMA–antibiotic spacer is placed in the joint to fill the dead space and to prevent shortening, which will make the revision arthroplasty difficult to perform. The spacer is a block with or without beads in the knee, and beads alone in the hip and shoulder. Appropriate antibiotics are administered systemically or locally via an implanted pump. Depending on the clinical course, the exchange arthroplasty is performed six weeks to one year later. Factors which mitigate for early exchange arthroplasty are: a rapid decrease in postoperative drainage; a precipitous fall in the erythrocyte sedimentation rate; and patient intolerance of a flail joint.

Case report

A 49 year old man presented 12 months following a knee arthroplasty, which was performed for osteoarthritis. Postoperatively, the patient had fallen and ruptured his patellar tendon. After repair of the tendon the skin over the tendon sloughed and a wound infection developed. Because of the persistent wound problems he had received three months of oral antibiotics and nine months of intravenous antibiotics. On presentation there was a draining sinus anteriorly; the patient could actively extend and flex the knee. Cultures from the sinus tract were negative. Antibiotics were stopped, and two weeks later a biopsy of the knee was performed. Cultures of biopsy material were positive for *Pseudomonas aeruginosa* and *Staphylococcus aureus* (Fig. 8.94). A pump was implanted, the prosthesis was removed, taking care to preserve the patellar tendon, and an antibiotic spacer was inserted into the defect. The outflow catheters from the pump were left in the defect and the incision was closed over large suction drains (Figs 8.95, 8.96).

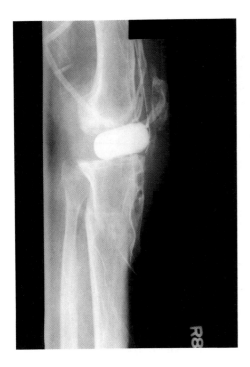

Figure 8.96

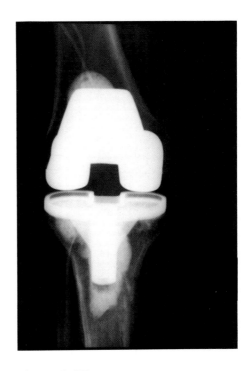

Figure 8.97

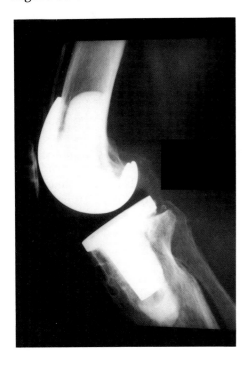

Figure 8.98

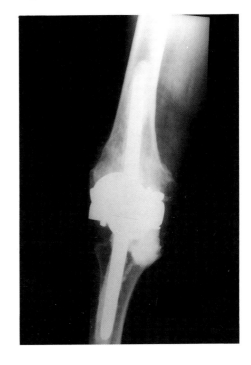

Figure 8.99

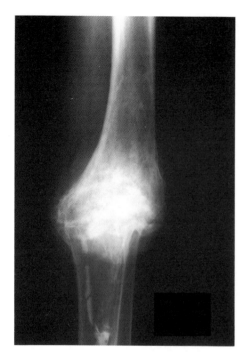

Figure 8.100

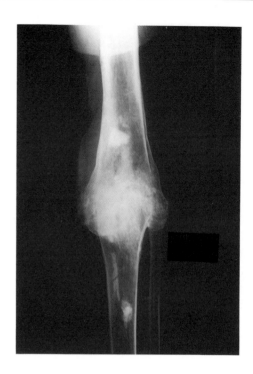

Figure 8.101

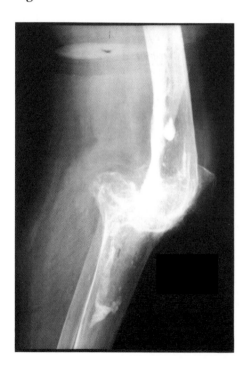

Figure 8.102

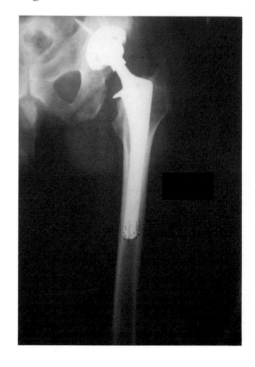

Figure 8.103

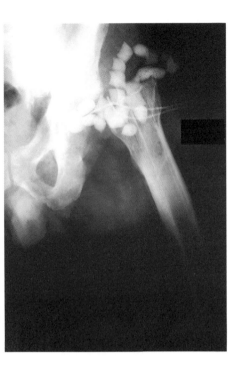

Figure 8.104

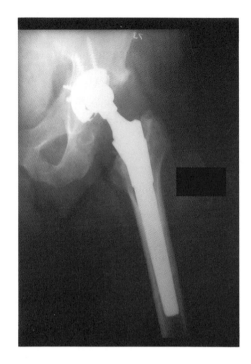

Figure 8.105

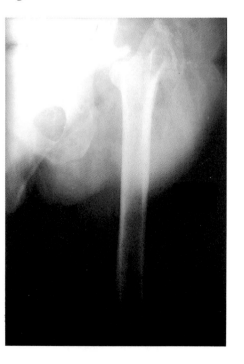

Figure 8.106

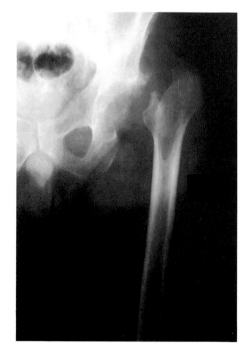

Figure 8.107

Postoperatively, the erythrocyte sedimentation rate dropped from 86 mm/h preoperatively to 18mm/h five weeks after débridement. Ten weeks after débridement a revision arthroplasty was performed (Figs 8.97, 8.98). The pump was removed two months after the revision arthroplasty. The patient is now 12 months post-therapy and continues to do well.

Removal of the prosthesis without reimplantation

Removal of the prosthesis without revision arthroplasty is considered when the patient is not ambulatory, and when it is not possible to eradicate the infection. A relative contraindication to reimplantation is when infection has recurred following a delayed exchange arthroplasty. In the past I have performed arthrodesis on knees in which revision arthroplasty was not possible. However, because of patient intolerance of a stiff knee, I now use an orthotic to stabilize the knee in the perioperative period. In most cases stability increases and the orthotic is eventually no longer required. Arthrodesis of the hip has not been necessary.

Case report

A 76 year old woman with rheumatoid arthritis developed a postoperative wound infection following a revision knee arthroplasty with a constrained prosthesis (Fig. 8.99). Cultures of wound drainage were positive for *Enterococcus*. The patient had been confined to a wheelchair for years. The prosthesis was removed, a spacer was not inserted because revision surgery was not contemplated, and the wound was closed over large suction drains (Fig. 8.100). Systemic antibiotics were administered for six weeks. The signs of infection rapidly diminished and disappeared, despite the fact that PMMA was left in the proximal tibia. The patient returned to her previous level of activity, using a double upright hinged knee brace for stability when transferring. Approximately one year following excision of the prosthesis, she felt that her knee was stable, and she independently discontinued the brace. There have been no further signs of infection and the femur and tibia have fused in 30° of flexion (Figs 8.101, 8.102).

Case report

A 63 year old man with a postoperative infection of his hip arthroplasty presented nine months after the onset of symptoms (Fig. 8.103). Cultures were positive for *Pseudomonas*, *Enterococcus* and *Staphylococcus epidermidis*. A pump was implanted, the prosthesis was excised, the defect packed with PMMA–antibiotic beads, the outflow catheters of the pump were left in the defect and the incision was closed over large suction drains (Fig. 8.104). The signs of infection quickly resolved. The pump was removed after three months, and a second prosthesis was inserted six months following the initial débridement (Fig. 8.105). Within six weeks cellulitis and drainage from the incision were present. Cultures were positive for *Staphylococcus epidermidis*. The prosthesis was excised, PMMA–antibiotic beads were not used, and the incision was closed over a large suction drain. (Fig. 8.106) There have been no further signs of infection, and the patient walks with a shoe lift, a crutch on the involved side, and a cane in the contralateral hand (Fig. 8.107).

References

1   Epps CH, Bryant DD, Coles MJ, et al, Osteomyelitis in patients who have sickle-cell disease. Diagnosis and prognosis, *J Bone Joint Surg* (1991) 73A:1281–1294.

2   Mallouh A, Talab Y, Bone and joint infection in patients with sickle cell disease, *J Pediatr Orthop* (1985) 5:158–162.

INDEX